Critical Care Foc

C000001501

11: Trauma

EDITOR
DR HELEN F. GALLEY
Senior Lecturer in Anesthesia and Intensive Care
University of Aberdeen

EDITORIAL BOARD
PROFESSOR NIGEL R. WEBSTER
Professor of Anesthesia and Intensive care
University of Aberdeen

DR PAUL G. P. LAWLER
Clinical Director of Intensive Care
University of Aberdeen

DR NEIL SONI
Consultant in Anesthesia and Intensive Care
Chelsea and Westminster Hospital

DR MERVYN SINGER
Reader in Intensive Care
University College Hospital, London

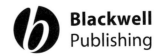

First published 2005

Library of Congress Cataloging-in-Publication Data

Trauma / editor, Helen F. Galley.
    p. ; cm. – (Critical care focus ; 11)
    Includes index.
    ISBN 0-7279-1694-7
    1. Traumatology. I. Galley, Helen F. II. Series: Critical care focus
series ; 11.
    [DNLM: 1. Wounds and Injuries. 2. Critical Care. 3. Spinal Injuries.
WO 700 T77315 2004]
    RD93.T67135 2004
    617.1–dc22
                                                        2004017386

ISBN 0727916947

A catalogue record for this title is available from the British Library

Set by Kolam Information Services Pvt. Ltd, Pondicherry, India
Printed and bound in India by Replika Press Pvt. Ltd

Commissioning Editor: Mary Banks
Development Editor: Claire Bonnett
Production Controller: Kate Charman

For further information on Blackwell Publishing, visit our website:
http://www.blackwellpublishing.com

Contents

Critical Care Focus Series

Also available:

H F Galley (ed) Critical Care Focus 1: *Renal Failure*, 1999.

H F Galley (ed) Critical Care Focus 2: *Respiratory Failure*, 1999.

H F Galley (ed) Critical Care Focus 3: *Neurological Injury*, 2000.

H F Galley (ed) Critical Care Focus 4: *Endocrine Disturbance*, 2000.

H F Galley (ed) Critical Care Focus 5: *Antibiotic Resistance and Infection Control*, 2001.

H F Galley (ed) Critical Care Focus 6: *Cardiology in Critical Issues*, 2001

H F Galley (ed) Critical Care Focus 7: *Nutritional Issues*, 2001

H F Galley (ed) Critical Care Focus 8: *Blood and Blood Transfusion*, 2002.

H F Galley (ed) Critical Care Focus 9: *The Gut*, 2002.

H F Galley (ed) Critical Care Focus 10: *Inflammation and Immunity*, 2003.

Contributors

Peter Andrews
Reader in Anaesthesia, Department of Clinical and Surgical Sciences, University of Edinburgh, UK and Honorary Consultant, Anaesthesia, Critical Care and Pain Medicine

Gareth Davies
Consultant in Accident and Emergency and Prehospital Care, the Royal London Hospital, London, UK

Matthew H. Fraser
Consultant in Spinal Injuries, The Queen Elizabeth Spinal Injuries Unit, Southern General Hospital, Glasgow, UK

Rod Little
Professor of Surgical Science, University of Manchester, UK and Emeritus Professor in Accident and Emergency Medicine (now retired)

David Lockey
Consultant, Anaesthesia & Intensive Care Medicine, Frenchay Hospital, Bristol, UK

Claude Martin
Professor of Anaesthesia and Intensive Care and Head of Anaesthesia and Intensive Care Department, Trauma Centre, Hopital Nord, Marseilles, France

James M. Ryan
Leonard Cheshire Professor in Conflict Recovery, University College, London, UK; Senior Lecturer in Trauma Care and Honorary Consultant in Accident and Emergency Medicine at UCL Hospitals Trust

Evelyn Teasdale
Consultant in Neuroradiology, Southern General Hospital, Glasgow, UK

Preface to the Critical Care Focus Series

The Critical Care Focus Series aims to provide a snapshot of current thought and practice, by renowned experts. The complete series should provide a comprehensive guide for all health professionals on key issues in today's field of critical care. The volumes are deliberately concise and easy to read, designed to inform and provoke. Most chapters are produced from transcriptions of lectures given at the Intensive Care Society meetings and represent the views of world leaders in their fields.

Helen F. Galley

1: Ballistic trauma

JAMES M. RYAN

Introduction

As a result of the increasing number of weapons in the UK, many missile wounds occur annually, resulting in death, significant morbidity and associated socio-economic costs. Penetrating missile wounds, injuries from blast phenomena and burns are the typical features of modern conventional war. Missile wounds are caused by bullets or by fragments from exploding shells, mines or bombs. Exposure to blast phenomena may result in unique and complex injury patterns.

Learning from history

There is a wealth of data on the cause and distribution of wounds in wars over the last 30 years. However, care is needed in interpretation as the number of wounded varies greatly depending on the particular war from which data came. For example, Vietnam data cover over 17 000 casualties, whereas in contrast, data from the Gulf War are restricted to only 63 casualties. Inclusion criteria are also very variable and many fail to record multiple injuries to different body systems in single casualties, and unfortunately these are the hallmark of modern war injury.

Although care is needed in interpreting the available data, given these anomalies, some broad statements concerning war injury can be made. The most common wounding agent in surviving casualties of war is a fragment wound, not a bullet wound, as many people may believe. In survivors, limb injuries are the most common, which simply reflects the lethal nature of hits to the trunk and head. However, the aim in modern war is to incapacitate, not kill, which has resulted in an increase in the number of multiple hits to multiple body regions in survivors. The reason for this tactic perhaps needs to be pointed out: large numbers of surviving casualties are a major financial and logistic burden on a nation engaged in war. There are many factors that govern the nature, severity and outcome of a war wound, including the type of weapon system used, the environment in which such weapons are deployed, e.g. desert or jungle terrain, and also the quality and timing of medical management. In short, there is no single description of an injury that merits the description "the war wound".

Classification of wounds

Wounding missiles can be classified as low-velocity (<2000 ft/sec) or high-velocity (>2000 ft/sec). However, these terms can be misleading; more important than velocity is the efficiency of energy transfer, which is dependent on the physical characteristics of the projectile, as well as kinetic energy, stability, entrance profile and the path travelled through the body, and the characteristics of the tissues injured. The management of most gunshot wounds and penetrating injuries can be adequately performed by clinicians without specialised training. A basic knowledge of wound ballistics will allow these patients to be treated successfully in their own locality, so there is no need for transfer to a major centre.

Wound ballistics

Any projectile has the potential to injure, whether it is a falling object, a piece of glass or a bullet. The energy of the projectile depends not only on the velocity but also on the mass and the distance travelled. The material the projectile is made of and its particular design profile can determine how, and therefore how much, energy is transferred to the target, and the nature of the damage. Both hard and soft tissues can be injured and one projectile can result in multisystem trauma.

Epidemiology of gunshot wounds

Civilians

The incidence of gunshot wounds in Europe is low. There is, of course, an increasing number of incidents but for an individual medical practitioner, experience of gunshot wounds is fairly minimal. However, certain centres, particularly in London, have been seeing an increasing number, with a change from pistol and shotgun injury to a wider range of weapon systems and more fragment wounds related to terrorism (Figures 1.1 and 1.2), forming part of a combined injury. This means that the spectrum of injuries seen in this country is wide, ranging from patients with a single gunshot wound to the other extreme – perhaps a patient with multiple

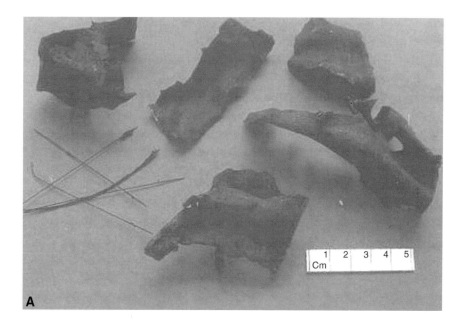

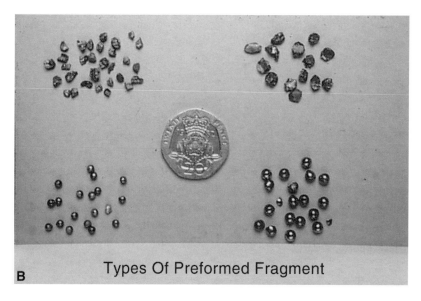

Figure 1.1 (A) Photograph showing typical fragments resulting from a terrorist bomb explosion. These are pieces of a litter bin in which the bomb had been placed. (B) Photograph showing military preformed fragments. These are small, regular in mass and shape and have low available energy. From the Department of Military Surgery, former Royal Army Medical College, Millbank, London (now closed).

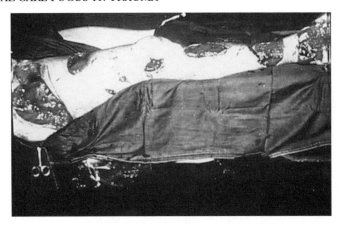

Figure 1.2 Victim of a terrorist bombing. Note multiple wounds that are heavily contaminated and of varying size and depth. From the Department of Military Surgery, former Royal Army Medical College, Millbank, London (now closed).

wounds, patients with explosive injuries, patients who are exposed to a flame front, patients who are exposed to a shock front and patients who may have a smoke inhalation injury in addition to multiple gunshot wounds.

A typical injury might be from a large handgun to the shoulder, when it is not clear whether the bullet has entered the chest and gone down through the diaphragm. Entry and exit wounds can "lie" and the bullet often does not move in a straight line through the body. This is one end of the spectrum, a single wound to a patient caused by a single bullet. Another end of the spectrum could be a patient caught in a terrorist attack, with multiple wounds, with many penetrating injuries likely to cause massive contamination, such that clinicians must deal not just with the penetrating physical injury to muscle but also with the possibility of serious sepsis.

Military

The epidemiology of injury in military conflict is of course quite different. The range of weapon systems capable of producing ballistic injury is massive, with a predominance of fragment wounds. In modern war, multiple wounds affecting multiple systems as part of a combined injury is seen. The number of casualties is high and even now there are still delays of several hours in getting patients from point of injury to the hospital, which itself causes problems.

Basic ballistics

The design characteristics of the firearm include the ability to maintain effectiveness after fragmentation, the tendency to deform, the amount of expansion and fragmentation on impact, and the generation of multiple projectiles. These factors can affect the wound channel size, the cavitation, the amount of foreign material entering the wound and the degree of thermal tissue damage. At one time the wound classification would be based on the weapon, where we would look at the individual injured and make a judgement based on the ballistics of the weapon and its ammunition. However, today, injuries are classified in terms of energy transfer – i.e. low-energy transfer or high-energy transfer – and we treat a patient exactly as we would any other patient with a physical injury.

Velocity and energy

The formula for kinetic energy is

$$KE = \frac{1}{2}MV(V_1^2 - V_2^2)$$

where KE is the available energy, M is the mass, and V_1 and V_2 are the velocities at entry and at exit, respectively.

Wounding missiles can be classified into low velocity (<600 m/s) or high velocity (>600 m/s). In general, bullets fired from handguns and most modern fragment munitions are propelled at low velocity, have low available energy (100–500 J) and result in low-energy transfer wounds. Missiles with high available energy (2000–3000 J) include high-velocity assault rifle bullets (>900 m/s) and some large fragments, and have potential to cause high-energy transfer wounds.

A bullet from a 38 mm handgun has a velocity of around 200 m/s and a 22 mm handgun around 400 m/s. Military rifles are typically high velocity, e.g. the AK47 having a velocity of 900 m/s (Figure 1.3). Shotguns are also low velocity at 400 m/s, but shotguns with solid slugs or fired from close range can also produce high-energy transfer injury. The bullets themselves can be low-energy transfer or high-energy transfer, which also affects the tissue damage. Military bullets are often jacketed, with small wound channels, capable of high velocity and accuracy, and which might cause tissue damage through cavitation. Low-energy transfer injuries are mainly from low-velocity bullets and include many handguns, perforating rifle bullets and also stab wounds. Other types of bullets can result in large wound channels through fragmentation, deformation and expansion. However, some modern high-performance handguns are now capable of firing high-velocity bullets with high available energy, and although this is very

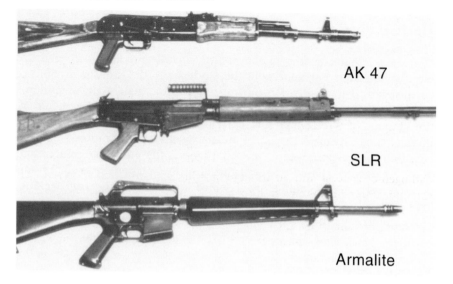

AK 47

SLR

Armalite

Figure 1.3 A selection of military assault rifles. From the Department of Military Surgery, former Royal Army Medical College, Millbank, London (now closed).

important in ballistic terms, it has very little relevance for clinicians. There are many other factors and we simply cannot make clinical judgements based on the velocity of a bullet.

Mechanisms of injury

By convention, missile wounds are described today in terms of energy transfer, not velocity as was the custom, recognising that velocity is merely one factor determining energy available and its transfer to tissues. Low-energy transfer wounds are characterised by injury confined to the wound track, and high-energy transfer wounds also cause local laceration and crush injury. However, they have, in addition, the potential to cause injury remote from the wound track associated with a phenomenon known as temporary cavitation.

Cavitation

The extent of cavitation depends upon the density and elasticity of the target organ or structure, and in certain circumstances is associated with injury some distance away from the missile wound track. Cavitation within solid organs such as the liver, spleen and kidney results in shattering and is associated with high morbidity and mortality. The extent of injury to bowel is variable and in general, the small bowel fares better than the colon, particularly if the latter is loaded with faeces. A similar injury in an elastic tissue such as the lung may result in quite modest injury. Cavitation injury to limbs is more complex and varied. Although voluntary muscle may merely stretch if injured in isolation, bone involvement tends to result in severe injury due to high-energy transfer with disruption of the missile and the bone itself generating secondary missiles. Extensive devitalisation of muscle happens frequently providing ideal conditions for the growth of pathogenic bacteria and all its complications. Nerves and blood vessels respond unpredictably with injury, ranging from minimal bruising to complete disruption. Within the closed skull there is, in addition, a rapid, high-pressure shock wave causing widespread disruption and injury at a distance. Thus, vital centres at the base of the brain may be injured by a wound of the cranium.

Other mechanisms

In addition to cavitation from high-energy transfer, injury from projectiles can result from several mechanisms, including direct laceration and crushing, damage from fragmentation or deformation and bacterial contamination. Although bullets do not become sterile as a result of discharge from a gun, most low-velocity gunshot wounds to soft tissue can be safely treated with local wound care. Complications of penetrating wounds include retained foreign bodies, development of infection, presence of fractures and associated damage to nerves, blood vessels or tendons. Special consideration should be given to crush injuries and subsequent potential for development of compartment syndrome.

Management of injury

Recommendations on an initial approach to patients presenting with penetrating trauma have been made by the American College of Emergency Physicians and are available in full at http://www2.us.elsevierhealth.com/scripts/om.dll/serve?retrieve=/pii/S019606449900164X&nav=full

Missile wounds of soft tissue

Management of soft tissue wounds is a formal procedure consisting of clearly defined stages. This is the part of early management most frequently neglected by clinicians with limited or no experience of war surgery. The entrance and exit wounds do not indicate the considerable damage that may have occurred to deeper structures and this can only be detected by full exploration. In limb wounds, exploration is followed by thorough wound excision, after which, with very few exceptions, the wound should be left open. All wounds treated by wound excision and left open should be inspected about 4–6 days after injury. Provided the wound looks healthy, delayed primary closure is indicated. This is done by interrupted suture, split skin graft or a combination of both.

Traumatic amputations

Traumatic amputations should be surgically tidied, completed at the lowest level possible and the skin left open for delayed primary closure. If there is much skin loss or if a limb is very swollen, split skin grafting may be used to effect wound closure in order to avoid skin tension. If, at the time of delayed primary closure, dead muscle is found, which is seen fairly commonly in traumatic amputation due to anti-personnel mines, the muscle should be excised and the wound left open for a further period before closure.

Missile wounds of the abdomen

Every penetrating and perforating missile wound of the abdomen should be explored by laparotomy. Before surgery, a nasogastric tube and a urinary catheter should be inserted. A full midline incision from xiphisternum to pubis is recommended and has the advantage of facilitating rapid access and extension laterally or into the chest where required. The commonest source of bleeding in survivors is from the small bowel mesentery, but major haemorrhage may come from the solid organs, such as liver or spleen, or from the major vessels. Haemorrhage must be controlled and careful examination should then be made of all the abdominal contents.

In all wounds of the stomach, the lesser sac must be opened to inspect the posterior gastric wall. Retroperitoneal haematoma in the region of the duodenum requires inspection of its posterior wall. Haematoma surrounding the retroperitoneal parts of the ascending and descending colon may also necessitate exploration, but non-expanding retroperitoneal haematomas over the kidneys are best left undisturbed.

Liver injuries

In around half of cases of hepatic injury that have survived to reach a surgical centre, bleeding has stopped and is not a problem at laparotomy.

Where bleeding still occurs, damage control techniques are particularly appropriate in a warfare setting. Manual compression and perihepatic packing are recommended, and may allow a patient to survive to reach a more sophisticated surgical facility. If these simple measures do not work, and provided that the operator is experienced, finger fracture with exposure of bleeding points followed by individual ligation, or more formal resection procedures, will be needed. However, these are rare eventualities. In all cases, generous drainage of the spaces surrounding the liver is important. The laparotomy wound should be closed using the mass closure technique. The missile entrance and exit wounds should be excised as described earlier and left open initially with a view to delayed primary closure at 4–6 days.

Missile wounds of the chest

Penetrating missile wounds of the chest are common in war and are associated with a high mortality. It is important to secure an airtight seal of open wounds of the chest to prevent a potentially fatal open pneumothorax and such injuries should be immediately followed by tube thoracostomy to prevent the accumulation of blood or air under tension. Once pulmonary function has been stabilised, missile entry and exit wounds should be excised. The opportunity should be taken to remove any retained foreign material, arrest haemorrhage (usually from an intercostal or internal mammary vessel) and to oversew or staple holes in the adjacent lung. On completion the pleural opening must be sealed either by direct pleural closure (often difficult) or by utilising overlying healthy soft tissue, and the wound left open for subsequent delayed primary closure.

In thoracoabdominal injuries, the thoracic component is treated by tube thoracostomy and the abdominal component by laparotomy through a midline incision. Formal thoracoabdominal incisions risk contamination of the chest cavity by faeces and should be avoided.

Missile wounds of the head

A penetrating high-energy transfer missile wound to the head is usually lethal. The management of penetrating low-energy transfer and tangential wounds depends initially on measures described in the primary survey and resuscitation phases. These will ensure a protected airway, adequate ventilation, and maintenance of blood pressure and perfusion pressure to permit oxygenation of the brain. Good radiographs are essential to identify and locate foreign bodies and bone fragments, and computerised tomography (CT) images are invaluable in planning surgical exploration. Wound excision should be carried out using gentle irrigation and suction to remove devitalised brain and bony fragments. Every effort, including the use of temporalis fascia or fascia lata, should be made to close overlying dura. The skin overlying the head and face is an exception to the delayed primary closure rule. Blood supply is excellent, allowing primary closure, which also serves to control blood loss from the scalp.

Intermittent positive pressure ventilation (IPPV) assists in the reduction of intracranial pressure by reducing brain swelling. Intracranial pressure transducers inserted through burr holes may be employed to monitor intracranial pressure in the postoperative phase.

Shotgun injuries

Accidents from large-bore shotguns are common and frequently lethal when injury is sustained at close range. It is never possible to retrieve all the shot and, indeed, to do so would result in unacceptable damage to uninjured soft tissues. Wound excision should be carried out on the major wound, particularly looking for wadding and plugs of clothing that have been driven into the tissue. Laparotomy is essential if shot is suspected to have penetrated an abdominal viscus. Retention of lead shot in the body can result in a dangerously high lead concentration, which should be monitored, although with time, the lead concentration will fall as a result of encapsulation of the lead pellets by fibrous tissue.

Antibiotics

Characteristics of wounds that may effect decisions regarding antibiotic therapy include wound location, presence of devitalised tissue, probable contamination, involvement of joint spaces, tendons or bones, and the presence of impaired host-immune responses. However, there is little evidence supporting the routine use of prophylactic antimicrobials, and antimicrobial use should be based on individual wounds at higher risk of infection.

Conclusion

The study of penetrating trauma has been largely in the military arena but such injuries often also present to civilian clinicians. A thorough understanding of the dynamic biomechanics of penetrating injuries in terms of injury to hard and soft tissue, depending on missile type, calibre and velocity is vital. Such information enables a comprehensive assessment of the acute and long-term treatment of patients with penetrating injuries. The management of most gunshot wounds and penetrating war injuries can be adequately performed by doctors without specialised training. A basic knowledge of wound ballistics and adherence to the principles outlined here will allow these patients to be treated successfully in their own locality, thus negating the necessity for transfer to a major centre. Failure to understand the underlying scientific basis of such injury has previously resulted in inappropriate management. Adherence to general management principles will reduce unnecessary mortality and morbidity.

Box 1.1 Summary: Dos and don'ts of handling missile injuries

Do:

- incise skin generously;
- incise fascia widely;
- identify neurovascular bundles;
- excise all devitalised tissue;
- remove all indriven clothing;
- leave wound open at end of surgery;
- dress wounds with fluffed gauze;
- record all injuries in the notes.

Don't:

- excise too much skin;
- practise keyhole surgery;
- repair tendons or nerves;
- remove attached pieces of bone;
- close the deep fascia;
- insert synthetic prostheses;
- pack the wound;
- close the skin.

Further reading

Coupland RM. *War Wounds of Limbs – Surgical Management*. Oxford: Butterworth-Heineman, 1993.

Galbraith KA. Combat casualties in the first decade of the 21st century – new and emerging weapon systems. *J R Army Med Corps* 2001 Feb;**147**:7–14.

Gugala Z, Lindsey RW. Classification of gunshot injuries in civilians. *Clin Orthop* 2003;**408**:65–81.

Husum H, Gilbert M, Wisborg T. *Save Lives, Save Limbs – Life Support for Victims of Mines, Wars and Accidents*. Malaysia: Third World Network, 2000.

Ryan JM, Rich NM, Dale RF, Morgans BT, Cooper GJ (eds). *Ballistic Trauma – Clinical Relevance in Peace and War*. London: Arnold, 1997.

2: The sympathetic response to trauma

ROD LITTLE

Introduction

The sympathetic system enables the body to be prepared for fear, flight or fight. Sympathetic responses include an increase in heart rate, blood pressure and cardiac output, a diversion of blood flow from the skin and splanchnic vessels to those supplying skeletal muscle, increased pupil size, bronchiolar dilation, contraction of sphincters and metabolic changes such as the mobilisation of fat and glycogen. The events that arise as a result of sympathetic nervous system activation are summarised in Boxes 2.1 and 2.2.

The sympathetic nervous system

Epinephrine (adrenaline) and norepinephrine (noradrenaline) are both catecholamines (biologically active amines) and are both synthesised from the essential amino acid phenylalanine by a series of steps, which includes the production of dopamine. The terminal branches of the sympathetic postganglionic fibres have varicosities or swellings. These swellings form the synaptic contact with the effector organ, and are also the site of synthesis and storage of norepinephrine. On the arrival of a nerve impulse, norepinephrine is released from granules in the presynaptic terminal into the synaptic cleft. The action of norepinephrine is terminated by diffusion from the site of action and reuptake into the presynaptic nerve ending, where it is inactivated by the enzyme monoamine oxidase in mitochondria or metaboled locally by the enzyme catechol-O-methyl-transferase. The action of norepinephine on a particular gland or muscle is excitatory in some cases, inhibitory in others.

The sympathetic nervous response is a very non-specific response to stress. This is because a single preganglionic neurone usually synapses with many postganglionic neurones, and the release of epinephrine from the adrenal medulla into the blood ensures that all the cells of the body will

---

Box 2.1 Activation of the sympathetic nervous system – effects on the cardiovascular system

- Vasoconstriction in most systemic arteries and veins (postjunctional α_1- and α_2-adrenoceptors).
- The overall cardiovascular response is increased cardiac output and systemic vascular resistance, resulting in an elevation in arterial blood pressure. Heart rate, although initially stimulated by norepinephrine, usually decreases due to activation of baroreceptors and vagal-mediated slowing of the heart rate.
- Increased heart rate and inotropy (β_1-adrenoceptor).
- Vasodilation in muscle and liver vasculatures at low concentrations (β_2-adrenoceptor); vasoconstriction at high concentrations (β_1-adrenoceptor-mediated).
- The overall cardiovascular response is increased cardiac output and a redistribution of the cardiac output to muscular and hepatic circulations with only a small change in mean arterial pressure.

Box 2.2 The release of norepinephrine

- Stimulates the heartbeat
- Raises blood pressure
- Dilates the pupils
- Dilates the trachea and bronchi
- Stimulates the conversion of liver glycogen into glucose
- Shunts blood away from the skin and viscera to the skeletal muscles, brain and heart
- Inhibits peristalsis in the gastrointestinal tract
- Inhibits contraction of the bladder and rectum

---

be exposed to sympathetic stimulation even if no postganglionic neurones reach them directly. Activation of the sympathetic nervous system can be stimulated in response to an enormous range of events – any situation that is psychologically or physiologically stressful, from anxiety to hypotension, fever, hypoxia and hypercapnia.

Sources of catecholamines

Circulating epinephrine and norepinephrine originate from two sources. Epinephrine is released by the adrenal medulla upon activation of preganglionic sympathetic nerves innervating this tissue. This activation occurs during times of stress (e.g. exercise, heart failure, haemorrhage, emotional stress or excitement, pain). Circulating norepinephrine also is released by the adrenal medulla (about 20% of its total catecholamine release is norepinephrine). Another source of norepinephrine is spillover from sympathetic nerves, particularly those innervating blood vessels. Normally, most of the norepinephrine released by sympathetic nerves is taken back by the nerves and some is also taken up by extraneuronal tissues where it is metabolised. A small amount of norepinephrine, however, diffuses into the blood and circulates throughout the body. At times of high sympathetic nerve activation, the amount of norepinephrine entering the blood increases dramatically.

The synthesis and storage of catecholamines in the adrenal medulla is similar to that of sympathetic postganglionic nerve endings, but due to the presence of an additional enzyme the majority of norepinephrine is converted to epinephrine. The adrenal medulla responds to nervous impulses in the sympathetic cholinergic preganglionic fibres by transforming the neural impulses into hormonal secretion. In situations involving physical or psychological stress, much larger quantities are released.

Catecholamine receptors

The actions of catecholamines are mediated by specific postsynaptic cell surface receptors. Pharmacological subdivision of these receptors into two groups (α and β) was first suggested by Ahlquist in 1948, based upon the effects of epinephrine at peripheral sympathetic sites. These have since been further subdivided on functional and anatomical grounds. Thus β_1-adrenoceptor-mediated effects in the heart (increased force and rate of contraction) have been differentiated from those producing smooth muscle relaxation in the bronchi and blood vessels (β_2-effects). Similarly, α-adrenoceptor-mediated effects such as vasoconstriction have been termed α_1-effects, to differentiate them from the feedback inhibition by noradrenaline on its own release from presynaptic terminals, which is mediated by α_2-adrenoceptors on the presynaptic membrane.

However, further research now shows that the classification is not as simple as this. For instance, many organs have both β_1- and β_2-adreno-ceptors (e.g. in the heart, there is one β_2-adrenoceptor to every three β_1-adrenoceptors). The receptors also show differing responses to epinephrine (adrenaline) and norepinephrine (noradrenaline). At β_1-adrenoceptors in the heart, epinephrine and norepinephrine appear to have an equal effect, whereas β_2-adrenoceptors in smooth muscle are more sensitive to circulating epinephrine than norepinephrine.

Assessment of the activation of the sympathetic nervous system

It is possible to measure circulating levels of norepinephrine in the plasma but it is important to remember that norepinephrine comes from nerve endings and not the adrenal medulla or the central nervous system, so plasma levels simply represent spillover from organs. Another consideration is the clearance rate of norepinephrine, bringing the conclusion that in fact plasma noradrenaline levels are at best difficult to interpret, and at worst mean very little. In a small study of six patients with sepsis there was no statistically significant difference in plasma norepinephrine levels during sepsis and after recovery, suggesting that circulating plasma norepinephrine is a poor indicator of sympathetic nervous system activity during septic illness (Figure 2.1) [1].

Perhaps a better approach is to measure urine levels of the metabolites normetepinephrine and metepinephrine, which gives to some extent, an integrated dynamic picture of activation. However, this approach, although better than plasma, has its difficulties. For example, non-metabolic clearance is not accounted for and there is also the age-old problem of variable urine excretion and clearance and also of simply obtaining accurate 24-h urine collections. Spillover and clearance of intravenous (i.v.) tritiated L-norepinephrine can also be measured in patients. Measurement of norepinephrine kinetics (clearance and spillover) may be a more accurate and direct assessment of sympathetic nervous system activity. In the study by Leinhardt et al.[1] norepinephrine kinetics were measured in six patients with intra-abdominal sepsis using ^{3}H-L-norepinephrine infused to achieve a plateau plasma concentration. The measurements were repeated in the same patients after they had recovered. Clearance and spillover were both significantly higher in the septic compared with the non-septic state (Figure 2.1). However, there are disadvantages: obviously the technique requires administration of a radioactive isotope and, in addition, since the distribution of the administered norepinephrine takes around 45–50 min, one must assume constant steady state conditions during this time. In a critically ill patient, that is a huge assumption. The plasma of levels of norepinephrine and the spillover/clearance did not correlate.

Phases of the sympathetic response to injury

There are two phases of the sympathetic response to injury. The early phase is the acute stress response. The acute phase of the response is followed by

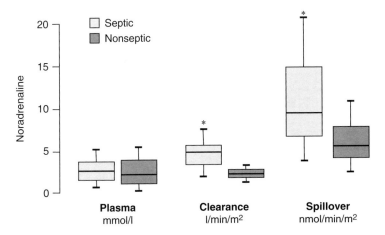

Figure 2.1 Plasma norepinephrine concentrations, norepinephrine spillover and norepinephrine clearance in six patients with intra-abdominal sepsis (septic) and in the same patients after resolution of sepsis (non-septic). Values are median, 25th and 75th percentile and ranges. ★ p = 0.028 compared to non-septic (Wilcoxon Signed Rank test). Redrawn with permission from data presented in Leinhardt DJ et al. [1].

the flow phase, characterised by hypermetabolism, insulin resistance and muscle wasting, commonly seen in patients in the intensive care unit (ICU). The sympathetic nervous system certainly contributes to increased metabolic rate but is not the only factor. Plasma catecholamine levels in the first 2 h after injury have been reported and were shown to correlate with the severity of injury, as shown by the injury severity score, and were certainly high enough to elicit biochemical metabolic responses [2]. So certainly, although plasma norepinephrine levels are a poor measurement, there is some evidence that acutely after injury the activity of the sympathetic nervous system is increased, and that may well have serious metabolic effect.

Plasma insulin levels also correlate with the injury severity score (Figure 2.2). However, although plasma glucose levels increase with catecholamine levels, plasma insulin is reduced. This may be due to the effect of plasma epinephrine on the secretion of insulin from the pancreas. Insulin then is universally low in patients who have high epinephrine levels and high glucose levels. In 40 patients with accidental injury norepinephrine and epinephrine concentrations were unrelated other than by a common rise with severity. Although plasma glucose concentrations rose after injury, this was related only to the plasma epinephrine concentration and not independently to injury severity. Plasma insulin concentrations were uniformly low, especially with respect to the hyperglycaemia, in patients with high plasma epinephrine concentrations. These relationships confirm the expected role of the sympathoadrenal system in the metabolic changes following injury in man [2].

17

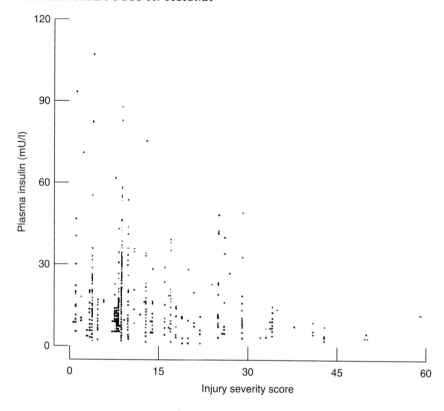

Figure 2.2 The relationship between plasma insulin concentrations and the injury severity score (ISS) in patients studied within 8 h of injury (n = 477). There is a significant negative correlation between insulin and ISS (p < 0.01, Kendall's Rank correlation). Reproduced with permission from Frayn KN et al. [3].

In the study by Frayn *et al.* [3] plasma insulin and glucose concentrations were measured in 504 patients within 8 h of injury, and related to the severity of injury as assessed by the injury severity score. Patients were classified as mildly, moderately, severely and very severely injured, as defined by injury severity scores of 0–6, 7–12, 13–29 and >30 respectively. An extremely wide range of insulin concentrations was found (2–141 mU/l) and most of the variability occurred at lower severities of injury. In very severely injured patients (injury severity score ≥ 30), insulin concentrations were suppressed, especially in relation to the hyperglycaemia in these patients (Table 2.1). The results bear out the idea that insulin secretion is usually acutely suppressed by epinephrine after severe injury, but in less severe injuries, the response is much less uniform. Patients being treated with α- or β-blockers had elevated glucose and insulin levels.

Table 2.1 Relationship between severity of injury and mean plasma glucose and insulin concentrations

	Injury severity score				
	0–6	7–12	13–29	> 30	αβ-block
Plasma glucose (mmol/l)	5.4	6.0	7.3	79.0	90.0
Plasma insulin (mU/l)	12.0	13.0	11.0	8.0	30.0

Reproduced with permission from Frayn KN *et al.* [3].

Catecholamines and thermogenesis

Increases in metabolic rate and core temperature are common responses to severe injury. Epinephrine is known to be thermogenic [4]; when given to volunteers it increases metabolic rate in a dose-dependent manner. There is also some evidence of a dose-dependent effect of epinephrine even in critical illness. Certainly the higher the epinephrine levels in some patients, especially burns patients, the higher their metabolic rates. The effects of β-blockade with propranolol were investigated during the first 3 weeks following burns [5]. The resting metabolic rate (RMR) of ten non-infected fasting burned patients (median [range] total burn surface area 28% [18–37]) was determined on four consecutive occasions by indirect calorimetry (open circuit hood system) as follows: after i.v. physiological saline, after i.v. propranolol infusion, after oral propranolol and also in control patients. All patients showed large increases in both RMR and in urinary catecholamine excretion. Oral and i.v. propranolol induced a significant decrease in RMR. Decreased lipid oxidation, but no change in carbohydrate and protein oxidation, was observed during propranolol administration. It was concluded that the magnitude of the decrease in energy expenditure suggests that β-adrenergic hyperactivity represents only one of the mediators of the hypermetabolic response to burn injury.

Wolfe *et al.* [6] investigated the hypothesis that the changes in metabolic rate are due to increases in substrate cycling. A substrate cycle is when opposing, non-equilibrium reactions catalysed by different enzymes, are operating simultaneously. At least one of the reactions must involve the hydrolysis of adenosine triphosphate (ATP). Thus, a substrate cycle liberates heat and increases energy expenditure, but there is no net conversion of substrate to product. In a study of 18 patients with severe burns who were in a hypermetabolic state and 18 volunteers as controls, stable-isotope tracers were used to measure substrate cycling in the pathways of glycolysis and gluconeogenesis, the triglyceride–fatty acid cycle. The total rates of triglyceride–fatty acid and glycolytic–gluconeogenic cycling were massively elevated in the patients. An infusion of the β-blocker propranolol in the patients greatly reduced triglyceride–fatty acid cycling but did not affect gluconeogenic–glycolytic cycling. These authors concluded that increased substrate cycling contributes to the increased thermogenesis and energy expenditure following severe burns, and that the increased triglyceride–fatty acid cycling is due to β-adrenergic stimulation [6].

Activation of stress-responsive pathways by the sympathetic nervous system after burn trauma has also been investigated. Burn trauma activates the stress-responsive proteins, p38 mitogen-activated protein kinase (MAPK), c-jun N H2-terminal kinase (JNK), and nuclear factor κB (NFκB); and p38 MAPK is an important mediator of cardiomyocyte tumour necrosis factor α (TNFα) secretion and cardiac dysfunction in burn trauma. Since burn trauma causes a rise in circulating catecholamine levels, it was hypothesised that the increased sympathetic activity may activate the p38 MAPK pathway after burn injury. In a recent study, Ballard-Croft et al. [7] determined whether the α_1-adrenergic receptor ligand phenylephrine could mimic burn trauma activation of p38 MAPK, JNK, and NFκB activation. In addition, the effect of the α_1-adrenergic receptor antagonist prazosin on activation of the stress response pathway by either phenylephrine or burn was determined. Rats were divided into seven groups: Group 1: untreated controls, Group 2: phenylephrine-treated controls, Group 3: phenylephrine -treated and prazosin-treated controls, Group 4: 40% burned, fluid resuscitated, Group 5: 40% burned, prazosin treated, fluid resuscitated, Group 6: sham burned, fluid resusciated and Group 7: sham-burned, prazosin treated, fluid resuscitated rats. Administration of phenylephrine to rats caused a significant activation of cardiac p38 MAPK/JNK and NFκB. Prazosin blocked phenylephrine-mediated changes in p38 MAPK/JNK activities. Burn injury activated cardiac p38 MAPK/JNK and NFκB, increased TNFα secretion by cardiomyocytes, and impaired cardiac function. Prazosin treatment in burns interrupted the burn-mediated signalling cascade, leading to a decrease in TNFα secretion by cardiomyocytes and preventing post-burn cardiac contractile dysfunction. It was concluded that burn trauma–related sympathetic activity activates the stress-responsive cascade, which regulates myocardial TNFα transcription/translation and results in cardiac contraction and relaxation defects.

Insulin resistance

There is no doubt that epinephrine is involved in the liberation of glucose by peripheral glycogenolysis, an effect which appears to be mediated by β-receptors. Insulin resistance can be elicited in animals and in volunteers by giving infusions of epinephrine and norepinephrine. Virkamaki et al. [8] investigated the role of catecholamines in acute endotoxin-induced alterations in glucose metabolism. Acute endotoxaemia was induced in rats by lipopolysaccharide (LPS) injection. Basal glucose turnover, in vivo insulin action on overall glucose utilisation, glycolysis, and glycogen synthesis were measured and the effects of α- or β-blockade or both were also determined. In the basal state, LPS induced hypotension and transient hyperglycaemia. These changes were associated with glycogen depletion in both skeletal muscle and liver, and increased basal glucose turnover. During hyperinsulinaemia, whole-body glucose disposal was decreased. This whole-body insulin resistance was characterised by decreased glycogen synthesis and glycogen synthase activity, but not by altered whole-body glycolysis. αβ-blockade abolished transient hyperglycaemia, increased basal glucose turnover and accelerated basal liver glycogen depletion but inhibited muscle glycogenolysis. However, αβ-blockade did not reverse the insulin resistance induced by endotoxin. These data suggest that catecholamines counteract the LPS-induced increase in basal glucose turnover and stimulate muscle glycogenolysis during acute endotoxaemia.

An alternative mechanism might involve counter-regulatory hormones. Patients with major injury or illness develop protein wasting, hypermetabolism and hyperglycaemia with increased glucose flux. To assess the role of elevated counter-regulatory hormones in this response, Gelfand et al. [9] infused cortisol ($6\,mg/m^2/h$), glucagon (4 ng/kg/min), epinephrine ($0.6\,\mu g/m^2/min$) and norepinephrine ($0.8\,\mu g/m^2/min$) simultaneously into five obese subjects for 72 h, whilst receiving only i.v. glucose (150 g/day) Figure 2.3. Four obese subjects received cortisol alone under identical conditions. The combined infusion maintained plasma hormone levels at those typical of severe stress for 3 days. This caused a sustained increase in plasma glucose, glucose production and total glucose flux, despite persistent hyperinsulinaemia. In contrast, RMR changed little. Urinary nitrogen excretion was doubled and remained increased by approximately 4 g/day, reflecting increased excretion of urea and ammonia. Concentrations of virtually all plasma amino acids decreased. Cortisol alone produced a smaller glycaemic response, an initially smaller insulin response and a delayed rise in nitrogen excretion. By day 3, however, nitrogen excretion and plasma insulin were the same as the combined group. Both infusions resulted in nitrogen wasting with modest increments in 3-methylhistidine and no significant change in leucine flux. The authors concluded that prolonged elevations of multiple stress hormones cause persistent hyperglycaemia, increased glucose turnover and increased nitrogen loss, but the sustained nitrogen loss is no greater than that produced by cortisol alone. In addition, glucagon, epinephrine and norepinephrine transiently augment cortisol-induced nitrogen loss and cause persistent hyperglycaemia.

However, circulating levels of the counter-regulatory hormones are less informative. In patients with sepsis or trauma, plasma levels of epinephrine and norepinephrine show very little change compared to controls. Cortisol is slightly increased and glucagon levels are very similar between controls and patients. Thus counter-regulatory hormones contribute to, but are probably not the sole mediators of, the massive nitrogen loss, muscle proteolysis and hypermetabolism seen in some clinical settings of severe stress.

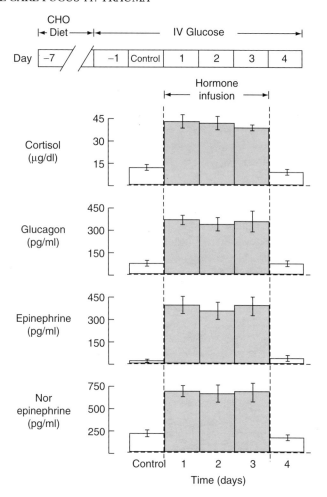

Figure 2.3 Effect of a 72-h infusion of cortisol, glucagon, epinephrine and norepinephrine on circulating levels of these counter-regulatory hormones in healthy obese subjects (n = 5). Values are mean and standard error of the mean. Reproduced with permission from Gelfand RA et al. [9].

Lipolysis and proteolysis

Lipolysis is also a feature of critical illness and injury. Catecholamines, again epinephrine acting at β-receptors, are able to liberate fatty acids from fat depots and have effects on the triglyceride–fatty acid cycle. However, this effect of adrenaline on the release of fatty acids from adipose tissue is sometimes not seen because of the sympathetic innervation of the vasculature of the adipose tissue, such that vasoconstriction masks the release of the fatty acids into the systemic circulation.

Septic and injured patients are catabolic although whether the sympathetic nervous system promotes proteolysis is unclear. In contrast, infusion of epinephrine actually reduces plasma amino acid concentrations. Thus there does not seem to be a very strong link between the sympathetic nervous system and protein catabolism, although there is some evidence that catecholamines have a role in protein synthesis through β_3-receptors as seen in the effect of anabolic agents used – or rather misused – by athletes.

Catecholamines and cytokines

There are close links between the cytokine network and the sympathetic nervous system, and stimulation of adrenergic and dopaminergic receptors can modulate the cytokine network [10]. Catecholamines alter the production of immune mediators in not only peripheral blood cells but also in various tissues such as liver, spleen, lung, heart, kidney and the skin. The sympathetic regulation of cytokines is highly dependent on the type of receptor stimulated. Whereas ligation of the α-adrenoreceptor is associated with predominantly immunostimulating effects, such as the induction of TNFα and interleukin-1β (IL-1β), stimulation of the β-adrenoreceptor usually has immunosuppressive consequences, such as inhibition of TNFα and IL-1β and induction of the anti-inflammatory cytokine, IL-10. Where both receptors are stimulated, e.g. by epinephrine, the β-adrenoreceptor-mediated effects usually dominate those induced by α-adrenoreceptor stimulation. Moreover, the adrenergic immunostimulation can be differentially regulated depending on the type of cell or tissue stimulated. Dopaminergic immunomodulation is dominated by immunosuppressive effects, via effects on IL-6, TNFα, IL-8 and adhesion molecules. Catecholamines also alter the number and function of neutrophils and lymphocytes depending on the type of receptor stimulated. Whereas β-adrenergic stimulation leads to lymphocytosis, α-adrenoreceptors mediate lymphocyte homing. Catecholamine-induced neutrophilia involves α_1-adrenoreceptor ligation and epinephrine increases the neutrophil respiratory burst. Up to now, most of the available data on catecholamine-induced immunomodulation were obtained in experimental settings, although it is clear that this system has important implications for the pathophysiology of the response to septic shock and trauma. Convincing evidence has been obtained that norepinephrine released non-synaptically from sympathetic axon terminals in the close proximity of immune cells is able to inhibit production of pro-inflammatory TNFα, interferon γ (IFNγ), IL-12, IL-1 and increase anti-inflammatory cytokines (IL-10) in response to LPS, suggesting fine-tuning control of the production of TNFα and other cytokines by sympathetic innervation under stressful conditions. These effects are mediated via β_2-adrenoceptors expressed on immune cells and coupled to cyclic adenosine monophosphate (cAMP) levels.

Catecholamines and cardiac arrest

Plasma catecholamine concentrations in cardiac arrest (ventricular fibrillation and asystole) are significantly higher than after myocardial infarction, and are also higher than those found after trauma [11]. The levels reached are well above those normally required to stimulate cardiac activity (Table 2.2). Some patients with myocardial ischaemia also had very high catecholamine levels. Despite an absence of electrocardiogram (ECG) evidence they all subsequently went into cardiac arrest and died, suggesting that very high circulating catecholamine levels might play a role in stimulating the arrhythmia that led to death.

Summary

Activation of the sympathetic nervous system is a cardinal feature of the acute response to injury. Activation is essential for many of the metabolical (e.g. mobilisation of energy stores for fight or flight) and physiological (e.g. cardiovascular changes elicited by hypovolaemia) responses to trauma. The assessment of the degree of activation, however, is not easy since there are limitations to the interpretation of changes in plasma levels of epinephrine (adrenaline) and norepinephrine (noradrenaline). A better, dynamic picture is given by measures of urinary excretion or turnover of, e.g. norepinephrine release and disposal, or direct recording of sympathetic efferent nerve activity. Despite the limitations of assessing sympathetic activity, direct relationships have been found between the extent of trauma and plasma catecholamines. The sympathetic nervous system has also been implicated in the catabolic or flow-phase response to critical illness and trauma. For example, adrenergic blockade reduces metabolic rate in burned patients. In addition, catecholamines, together with the other counter-regulatory hormones cortisol and glucagon, may in part mediate insulin resistance. Possibly the most important metabolic consequences of the catecholamines relate to their interactions with cytokines.

Table 2.2 Mean plasma concentrations of epinephrine, norepinephrine and dopamine after acute myocardial infarction, cardiac arrest and in healthy controls

	Epinephrine	Norepinephrine (nmol/l)	Dopamine
Myocardial infarction ($n = 11$)	1.5	5.8	0.22
Cardiac arrest			
ventricular fibrillation ($n = 26$)	14.9	26.9	1.3
asystole ($n = 25$)	16.3	26.7	2.0
Healthy controls ($n = 12$)	0.3	2.0	0.06

Reproduced with permission from Little RA et al. [11].

References

1 Leinhardt DJ, Arnold J, Shipley KA, Mughal MM, Little RA, Irving MH. Plasma NE concentrations do not accurately reflect sympathetic nervous system activity in human sepsis. *Am J Physiol* 1993;**265**:E284–8.
2 Frayn KN, Little RA, Maycock PF, Stoner HB. The relationship of plasma catecholamines to acute metabolic and hormonal responses to injury in man. *Circ Shock* 1985;**16**:229–40.
3 Frayn KN, Maycock PF, Little RA, Yates DW, Stoner HB. Factors affecting the plasma insulin concentration shortly after accidental injury in man. *Arch Emerg Med* 1987;**4**:91–9.
4 Wilmore DW, Long JM, Mason AD Jr, Skreen RW, Pruitt BA Jr. Catecholamines: mediator of the hypermetabolic response to thermal injury. *Ann Surg* 1974;**180**:653–69.
5 Breitenstein E, Chiolero RL, Jequier E, Dayer P, Krupp S, Schutz Y. Effects of beta-blockade on energy metabolism following burns. *Burns* 1990;**16**:259–64.
6 Wolfe RR, Herndon DN, Jahoor F, Miyoshi H, Wolfe M.Effect of severe burn injury on substrate cycling by glucose and fatty acids. *N Engl J Med* 1987; **317**:403–8.
7 Ballard-Croft C, Maass DL, Sikes P, White J, Horton J. Activation of stress-responsive pathways by the sympathetic nervous system in burn trauma. *Shock* 2002;**18**:38–45.
8 Virkamaki A, Yki-Jarvinen H. Mechanisms of insulin resistance during acute endotoxemia. *Endocrinology* 1994;**134**:2072–8.
9 Gelfand RA, Matthews DE, Bier DM, Sherwin RS. Role of counterregulatory hormones in the catabolic response to stress. *J Clin Invest* 1984;**74**:2238–48.
10 Bergmann M, Sautner T. Immunomodulatory effects of vasoactive catecholamines. *Wien Klin Wochenschr* 2002;**114**:752–61.
11 Little RA, Frayn KN, Randall PE, Stoner HB, Yates DW, Laing GS, Kumar S, Banks JM. Plasma catecholamines in patients with acute myocardial infarction and in cardiac arrest. *Q J Med* 1985;**54**:133–40.

3: Immune responses after trauma and haemorrhagic shock

CLAUDE MARTIN

Introduction

Death after multiple trauma occurs either immediately at the scene of the accident, or within hours after the event when patients are hospitalised. These fatalities are mainly due to the severity of injury or to direct complications from the primary injury. However, many patients survive the primary insult but die later after days or even weeks because of complications in remote organ systems not necessarily affected by the primary trauma. In the latter group, most patients die of adult respiratory distress syndrome (ARDS) and/or multiple organ failure syndrome that are thought to have one common pathophysiological background. This article discusses the role of immune function in the late death after trauma and the contribution of haemorrhage to immune responses.

Morbidity and mortality after trauma

We know that in Europe trauma is a major cause of death and if one considers the first three decades of life, trauma certainly ranks as the fourth leading cause of death in young people. Early mortality after trauma is commonly due to very severe neurological damage or to uncontrolled haemorrhage. Among those patients who survive the initial insult itself, many die from uncontrolled systemic inflammatory response syndrome (SIRS), subsequent infection and sepsis, or ARDS and multiple organ failure. It can often be days and even weeks after the initial insult.

In multiple trauma patients, head injury accounts for approximately 50%, haemorrhage for approximately 10–15%, and ARDS, multiple organ failure and sepsis account for approximately 30–35% of deaths. The occurrence rate of multiple organ failure after multiple traumas varies from 21% to 47% and the mortality rate within this group varies from 20% to 30%, depending on the patient populations studied and definitions used.

The contribution of trauma and haemorrhage to immune responses

Inflammation is characterised by interplay of cytokines. Combinations of types of injury may dictate the subsequent immune and inflammatory responses. A number of clinical studies have shown that multiple and severe traumas cause immunosuppression and increase the susceptibility to subsequent sepsis and organ failure. However, because there is a close relationship between trauma and haemorrhage in humans, it is difficult to dissociate the effects of tissue trauma versus haemorrhage on immunity in the clinical setting. To determine whether haemorrhage without major tissue trauma can itself produce immunosuppression, the effect of haemorrhage on lymphocyte responses to T-cell mitogen in endotoxin-resistant mice was measured in the study by Stephan *et al.* [1]. The mice were bled to achieve a mean blood pressure of 35 mmHg, which was maintained at that level for 1 h, after which resuscitation took place. Determination of proliferative responses to mitogen stimulation showed that marked immunosuppression occurred at day 1 and lasted for at least 5 days following haemorrhage. Another group of mice was additionally made septic 3 days after haemorrhage and resuscitation. The mortalities in the haemorrhage only and haemorrhage plus sepsis groups was 58% and 100% respectively, showing that depression of cellular immunity occurred following simple haemorrhage despite adequate resuscitation, which enhanced the susceptibility to sepsis.

However, the scenario in such animal studies is not the same as the one we observe in our patients. The magnitude of the immune response is variable in the trauma patient, depending on individual circumstances (Figure 3.1). If the patient has an adequate response, i.e. an effective and appropriate response and no immune suppression, this patient is unlikely to

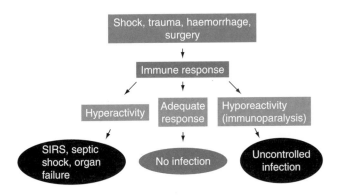

Figure 3.1 Schematic diagram showing how the quality of the immune response determines the outcome from trauma and haemorrhage.

27

develop an infection and will probably have an uneventful course in the intensive care unit (ICU). However, an inadequate immune response may not occur in some patients. Some trauma patients may manifest exaggerated cytokine production – a hyperactive response – and this finding has been attributed to repeated bacterial stimulation during septic episodes and to stimulation by trauma-induced release of activators of the inflammatory cascade. Hyporeactivity on the other hand, or the so-called immune paralysis, can lead to uncontrolled infection and subsequent death [2].

Immune responses and outcome from trauma

Inflammation

There is a very well-known uncontrolled hyperinflammatory response that leads to SIRS, septic shock and probably the development of multiple organ failure and ultimately death, characterised by release of pro-inflammatory mediators. Cytokines are commonly classified as pro- or anti-inflammatory. Interleukin-1 (IL-1), tumour necrosis factor α (TNFα), interferon-γ (IFNγ), IL-12, IL-18 and granulocyte-macrophage colony stimulating factor (GM-CSF) are described as pro-inflammatory cytokines whereas IL-4, IL-10, IL-13, IFNα and transforming growth factor β (TGFβ) are recognised as anti-inflammatory cytokines. However, some cytokines such as IL-6 and IL-8 have both pro- and anti-inflammatory roles and the classification may be simplistic rather than simple. The inflammatory response plays a key role in the development of (remote) cell and organ dysfunction, which is the basis of ARDS and multiple organ failure.

Some years ago Roumen et al. [3] described the course of serum cytokine levels in three groups of patients: those with multiple trauma (n = 28), those in haemorrhagic shock after a ruptured abdominal aortic aneurysm (n = 20), and those undergoing elective aneurysm repair (n = 18). They studied the relationship of these cytokines to the subsequent development of ARDS and multiple organ failure. Twenty-two patients died, 15 within 48 h, and seven after several weeks as a result of ARDS and/or multiple organ failure. These non-survivors had significantly higher admission plasma TNFα and IL-1β levels than the survivors had. Those with ARDS and/or multiple organ failure had different cytokine patterns in the early post-injury phase. In addition, IL-6 correlated with the organ failure score during the study period. The authors concluded that in the early post-injury phase, higher concentrations of cytokines are associated with both an increased mortality rate and with an increased risk of subsequent ARDS and organ failure. These data therefore support the concept that these syndromes are caused by an overwhelming autodestructive and uncontrolled hyperactive inflammatory response.

In a later study [4], the patterns of evolution of TNFα and IL-6 were studied in 25 patients with septic shock and 60 patients with multiple traumas, of whom eight had been resuscitated from haemorrhagic shock (Figure 3.2). High concentrations of circulating TNFα and IL-6 were found in patients with septic shock, and high IL-6 concentrations, but normal TNFα concentrations, were found in trauma patients. Non-surviving septic shock patients had higher TNFα and IL-6 concentrations at study entry than non-surviving trauma patients, and these remained high during the study period. IL-6 concentrations were higher throughout the study period in septic shock patients than in trauma patients. In septic shock patients, changes in both TNFα and IL-6 correlated with outcome, but neither TNFα nor IL-6 values were related to outcome of trauma patients. However, increased IL-6 values were an indicator of the development of a nosocomial infection in trauma patients. In summary, in septic shock patients, high amounts of circulating TNFα and IL-6 were found and correlated with fatal outcome. In trauma patients, including those

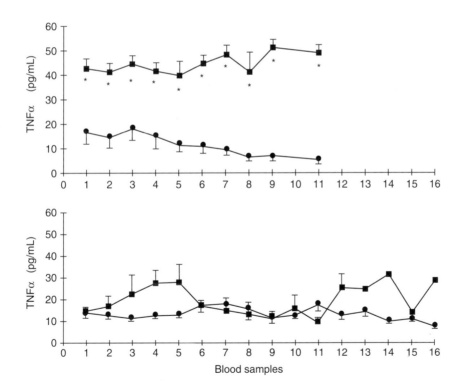

Figure 3.2 Circulating tumour necrosis factor α (TNFα) concentrations in patients with septic shock (top panel) and patients with trauma (lower panel). Squares, non-survivors; circles, survivors. * = significantly higher than in survivors. Reproduced with permission from Martin C et al. [4].

patients resuscitated from haemorrhagic shock, cytokines were lower and not related to outcome. This finding suggests that the immuno-inflammatory cascade is more activated in septic shock than in multiple trauma patients.

Immune paralysis

The term immune paralysis has been given to hyporeactive immune responses (immune suppression) after trauma, haemorrhage, burns, surgery or sepsis characterised by anti-inflammatory responses. HLA-DR expression may affect antigen presentation by monocytes and macrophages, and low HLA-DR expression is recognised as a good marker of immune depression and of increased risk of infection. In a study by Hershman et al. [5], trauma patients who developed sepsis took much longer for their HLA-DR expression to return to normal, and in the patients who did not survive, expression never returned to normal. The study showed that monocyte HLA-DR antigen expression correlated directly with the clinical course and was able to distinguish those patients who survived severe trauma from those who developed sepsis and those who died.

In a mouse model, Zellweger et al. [6] showed that traumatic injury in the form of a midline laparotomy combined with haemorrhage produces a more protracted impairment in cell-mediated immunity (determined as cytokine release) than laparotomy or haemorrhage alone. Also using a mouse model, Wichman et al. [7] found that bone fracture followed by haemorrhagic shock further depressed splenocyte proliferation and splenocyte IL-2 and IL-3 release as well as IL-1 release. Since bone injury coupled with haemorrhagic shock produces more severe depression of immune functions than haemorrhage alone, bone injury appears to play a contributory role in further depressing immune functions in trauma patients who experience major blood loss.

Several studies have indicated that simple haemorrhage produces a profound depression of cell-mediated immunity, thereby contributing to an enhanced susceptibility to septic challenge in the host. However, it remains unknown whether or not macrophage cytotoxic capacity is altered after haemorrhage. To study this, mice were subjected to haemorrhage and then adequately resuscitated in a study by Ayala et al. [8]. Cytotoxicity was assessed in peritoneal macrophages, splenic macrophages and Kupffer cells. It was found that peritoneal and splenic macrophages from haemorrhaged animals had reduced cytotoxic capacity, whereas cytotoxic capacity was enhanced in Kupffer cells. Kupffer cells were also able to maintain their capacity to release TNF and IL-1.

We know that macrophage function is very important in the mechanism of the fight against infection after trauma and haemorrhage. Antigen presentation is a very complex process by which the cell is able to express antigen on the cell surface in a form that is capable of being recognised by T cells. The antigen is degraded into small peptides either in association with MHC class II for presentation to T helper (Th) cells, or with MHC class I as a target for cytotoxic T (Tc) cells.

Depression of macrophage antigen presenting capacity contributes to the depression of cell-mediated immunity after trauma and increases the susceptibility to infection. Decreased expression of monocyte HLA-DR expression is more common in trauma patients who develop sepsis than those who do not. Docke et al. [9] reported that many patients die late after trauma with signs of opportunistic infections accompanied by downregulation of their monocyte HLA-DR expression and reduced ability to produce TNFα in response to LPS in vitro. This phenomenon of monocyte deactivation associated with fatal outcome shows similarities to experimental depression of monocyte function induced by pretreatment with anti-inflammatory cytokines such as IL-10 and TGFβ. In mice with haemorrhagic shock, decreased splenocyte and T-cell proliferation was associated with enhanced release of IL-10 but IL-10 release by macrophages was not elevated. While no changes were seen in systemic plasma levels of IL-10, the role of IL-10 as a localised immunosuppressant was demonstrated by the ability of IL-10 monoclonal antibody to restore T-cell proliferation following haemorrhage. Such a mechanism of cell-mediated immunosuppression may directly contribute to the decreased capacity to ward off infectious challenge seen following haemorrhage and trauma.

T cells show an immediate functional paralysis after trauma, the degree and length of which seem to be proportional to injury severity. Some 15 years ago Mosmann [10] noted that under certain conditions, T-helper lymphocytes can be subdivided into two functionally distinct, highly polarised subsets, termed Th1 and Th2, depending on their pattern of cytokine secretion and related functional activities (Figure 3.3). Exposure of naive Th cells to certain antigens and cytokines causes conversion to either the Th1 or the Th2 phenotype. Th1 cells produce IL-2 and IFNγ and initiate cellular immunity. Th2 cells secrete IL-4 and IL-10 and stimulate production of certain antibodies. Conversion to the Th1 phenotype is facilitated by IL-12, and conversion to the Th2 phenotype is promoted by IL-4. Th1 cells are further defined by their production of TNFβ (lymphotoxin). Th2 cells are further defined by their production of IL-5, IL-6, IL-9 and IL-13. Several other proteins are secreted by both Th1 and Th2 cells, including IL-3, TNFα and GM-CSF. It is believed that serious injury causes conversion of Th cells to the Th2 as opposed to the Th1 phenotype rather than generalised Th suppression. It is generally considered that Th1 predominance is associated with cell-mediated responses, which are most beneficial to recovery after surgery [11]. Th2 responses are generally anti-inflammatory and linked to immune paralysis. A shift to Th2-dominated phenotypes increases the risk for postburn infection and the studies by Zedler et al. [12,13] confirmed that major burns induce a significant shift

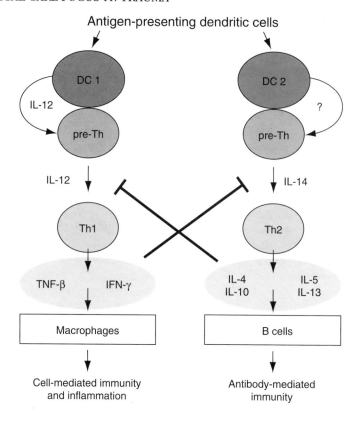

Figure 3.3 Diagram of the cross-regulation of T helper (Th) cell subsets. See text for explanation.

of cytokine response in the Th2 direction. In a pilot study Th subsets were measured using intracellular cytokine expression in lymphocytes from ten patients with severe sepsis, seven APACHE II score-matched non-septic critically ill control patients, and ten healthy subjects [14]. The Th1/Th2 ratio was significantly lower in patients with sepsis than both non-septic controls and healthy subjects and was due to both a decrease in Th1 cells and an increase in Th2 cells. It was concluded that in patients with sepsis, Th2 antibody-mediated (humoral) immune responses predominate, which may lead ultimately to immunosuppression.

Patients with serious traumatic injury and major burns and an animal model of burn injury were studied to determine the effect of injury on the production of cytokines typical of the Th2 lymphocyte phenotype as opposed to the Th1 phenotype [15]. Peripheral blood mononuclear cells from burn and trauma patients produced less IFNγ, the index cytokine of Th1 cells, than those from healthy subjects. However, production of IL-4, the index cytokine of Th2 cells, by patients' cells was increased.

Also studied was a mouse model of 20% burn injury known to mimic the immune abnormalities seen in humans with burns [15]. Burned mice were compared with sham-burn controls and attention was focused on day 10 after burn injury – a time when IL-2 production and resistance to infection are highly suppressed. Also burn and sham-burn animals were treated *in vivo* with IL-12 and after septic challenge (caecal ligation and puncture) performed on day 10 after burn injury. Splenocytes from mice 10 days after burn injury, when compared with sham-burn controls, showed diminished production of IL-2 and IFNγ. However, burn splenocytes produced more IL-4 and IL-10. Splenocyte production of IL-12 was also reduced after burn. *In vivo* IL-12 treatment of burn animals decreased mortality from sepsis after injury from 85% to 15% and increased splenocyte IFNγ production to above normal levels. These studies showed that a switch to Th2 predominance was seen after injury in patients, and in a complimentary mouse model, increased mortality from subsequent sepsis was reduced by treatment with IL-12, which encourages a change to Th1.

Apoptosis

Apoptosis or programmed cell death is really a phenomenon where cells are programmed to die at a particular point, e.g. during embryonic development. It is a continuous process of destruction of non-functional cells. It is a physiological process whereby the body disposes of unwanted cells by self-destruction and is the ultimate defence against damaged cells. There are several pathways leading to programmed cell death, and apoptosis can be defined as "gene-directed cellular self-destruction" and is distinct from necrosis. Apoptosis removes cells without causing inflammation, unlike necrosis. Increased signals for apoptosis leading to increased loss of cells may contribute to immune suppression by removing immunologically active cells.

Apoptosis in the organs of rats in the early stages after polytrauma combined with shock was recently studied by Guan *et al.* [16] in a rat model. Six groups (n = 6) were studied: (1) normal control, (2) sham-operation, (3) single haemorrhagic shock, (4) two-site trauma with shock, (5) four-site trauma with shock, and (6) six-site trauma with shock. Shock was performed by blood withdrawal and maintained for 1 h. Polytrauma was performed by clamping different sites of limbs to cause fractures at both femurs, at femurs and tibias, and at femurs, tibias and humeri. Apoptosis was assessed as the percentage of DNA fragmentation. At 6 h after resuscitation, the percentages of DNA fragmentation in thymus, spleen, liver, lung and intestine all increased with the severity of trauma. It was shown by morphological examination that the majority of apoptotic cells lay in the cortex of thymus, in the growth centre of white pulp of spleen, in the border area of hepatic lobule and the portal area of liver, and

33

at the base of crypts of intestine. In lung, multiple kinds of cells, including alveolar epithelial cells, vascular endothelial cells and polymorphonuclear neutrophils, showed evidence of apoptosis. The authors concluded that apoptosis was induced in thymus, spleen, liver, lung and intestine in early stage after polytrauma combined with shock. The defensive mechanisms could be affected by cell loss, which may contribute to the development of multiple organ failure.

Conclusion

Many patients survive primary trauma but die later after days or even weeks because of complications in remote organ systems not necessarily affected by the primary trauma. The immune responses after trauma and haemorrhage have profound effects on subsequent susceptibility to infection, organ failure and late death.

References

1 Stephan RN, Kupper TS, Geha AS, Baue AE, Chaudry IH. Hemorrhage without tissue trauma produces immunosuppression and enhances susceptibility to sepsis. *Arch Surg* 1987;**122**:62–8.
2 Cavaillon J-M, Galley HF. Immunoparalysis. In: Galley HF, ed. Critical Care Focus 10: *Inflammation and Immunity*. London, BMJ Books. 2003, pp. 1–17.
3 Roumen RM, Hendriks T, van der Ven-Jongekrijg J, Nieuwenhuijzen GA, Sauerwein RW, van der Meer JW, Goris RJ. Cytokine patterns in patients after major vascular surgery, hemorrhagic shock, and severe blunt trauma. Relation with subsequent adult respiratory distress syndrome and multiple organ failure. *Ann Surg* 1993;**218**:769–76.
4 Martin C, Boisson C, Haccoun M, Thomachot L, Mege J. Patterns of cytokine evolution (tumor necrosis factor-alpha and interleukin-6) after septic shock, hemorrhagic shock, and severe trauma. *Crit Care Med* 1997;**25**:1813–9.
5 Hershman MJ, Cheadle MJ, Wellhausen SR, Davidson PF, Polk HC Jr. Monocyte HLA-DR antigen expression characterizes clinical outcome in the trauma patient. *Br J Surg* 1990;77:204–7.
6 Zellweger R, Ayala A, DeMaso CM, Chaudry IH. Trauma-hemorrhage causes prolonged depression in cellular immunity. *Shock* 1995;**4**:149–53.
7 Wichmann MW, Zellweger R, DeMaso CM, Ayala A, Williams C, Chaudry IH. Immune function is more compromised after closed bone fracture and hemorrhagic shock than hemorrhage alone. *Arch Surg* 1996;**131**:995–1000.
8 Ayala A, Perrin MM, Wang P, Ertel W, Chaudry IH. Hemorrhage induces enhanced Kupffer cell cytotoxicity while decreasing peritoneal or splenic macrophage capacity. Involvement of cell-associated tumor necrosis factor and reactive nitrogen. *J Immunol* 1991;**147**:4147–54.
9 Docke WD, Randow F, Syrbe U, Krausch D, Asadullah K, Reinke P, Volk HD, Kox W. Monocyte deactivation in septic patients: restoration by IFN-gamma treatment. *Nat Med* 1997;**3**:678–81.

10 Mosmann TR. Cytokine secretion patterns and cross-regulation of T cell subsets. *Immunol Res* 1991;**10**: 183–8.

11 Le Cras AE, Galley HF, Webster NR. Spinal but not general anesthesia increases the ratio of T helper 1 to T helper 2 cell subsets in patients undergoing transurethral resection of the prostate. *Anesth Analg* 1998;**87**:1421–5.

12 Zedler S, Faist E, Ostermeier B, von Donnersmarck GH, Schildberg FW. Postburn constitutional changes in T-cell reactivity occur in CD8+ rather than in CD4+ cells. *J Trauma* 1997;**42**:872–80.

13 Zedler S, Bone RC, Baue AE, Donnersmarck GH, Faist E. FACS T-cell reactivity and its predictive role in immunosuppression after burns. *Crit Care Med* 1999;**27**:66–72.

14 Ferguson NR, Galley HF, Webster NR. T helper cell subset ratios in patients with severe sepsis. *Intensive Care Med* 1999;**25**:106–9.

15 O'Sullivan ST, Lederer JA, Horgan AF, Chin DH, Mannick JA, Rodrick ML. Phenotype and diminished interleukin-12 production associated with decreased resistance to infection. *Ann Surg* 1995;**222**:482–90.

16 Guan J, Jin DD, Jin LJ, Lu Q. Apoptosis in organs of rats in early stage after polytrauma combined with shock. *J Trauma* 2002;**52**:104–11.

4: Management of acute spinal injury

MATTHEW H. FRASER

Ludwig Guttman was a neurosurgeon whose goal was to provide athletes with disabilities the opportunity to compete at the same international level as athletes without disabilities. He described spinal cord injury as the most devastating injury known to mankind. Although the acute care of a spinal injury may influence subsequent recovery, a patient with spinal cord injury needs lifelong management. Traumatic spinal cord injury is often associated with brain injury, and effects on respiratory and cardiovascular function require initial management in the intensive care unit (ICU). Complications may include respiratory failure, atelectasis, pneumonia, neurogenic shock, autonomic dysreflexia (Box 4.1), venous thromboembolism and sepsis. However, although such complications can be managed, improving neurological outcome is a bigger challenge.

Epidemiology of spinal cord injury

Spinal cord injuries are most common in young men, particularly those aged around 30 years. About 10–15 per million of the population in the UK have a spinal cord injury and this is around 850 per annum. The mortality rate at the Queen Elizabeth National Spinal Injuries Centre (QENSIC) in Glasgow is overall nine patients per annum (5.3%) and most of these deaths occur in patients aged over 70 years. These figures are similar to those in other units.

The commonest cause of spinal cord injury presenting to QENSIC is road traffic accidents, followed by domestic and industrial falls and sporting injuries. Self-harm and assault account for only 10% of cases. Around 5–10% of patients with a cervical spinal cord injury are unconscious at presentation.

Box 4.1 Autonomic dysreflexia

Definition
- Life-threatening syndrome in spinal cord injury above T6
- Most common in quadriplegia
- Pathological response to pain or other noxious stimuli
- Characterised by hypertension, bradycardia and vasodilation above the level of the cord injury

Pathophysiology
- Distention/contraction of bladder/bowel, stimulation of skin or pain receptors triggers a sympathetic response (from intact autonomic reflex arc) below the level of the lesion.
- Catecholamines cause vasoconstriction and hypertension.
- Hypertension stimulates baroreceptors in the carotid sinus, aorta and cerebral vessels, causing stimulation of parasympathetic nervous system in attempt to restore normal blood pressure. Heart rate decreases.
- Vasoconstriction below the level of the cord injury causes the hypertension to persist.

Signs and symptoms
- Vasoconstriction causes hypertension and decreased peripheral circulation below the level of the cord injury.
- Vasodilation above the level of the cord injury causes facial flushing, head-ache, nasal congestion, blurred vision, nausea and diaphoresis.
- Inhibition causes bradycardia.

Causes
- Bladder distention
- Bladder infection
- Faecal impaction
- Cold or draught on the skin
- Pressure sores
- Sharp objects pressing on skin

Treatment
- Find and remove cause.
- Treat hypertension.
- If faecal impaction is the cause, blood pressure control is the priority. Topical anaesthetic agents should be applied rectally until the blood pressure is controlled.

Prevention
- Maintain meticulous bowel routine.
- Monitor bladder catheter for obstruction.
- Inspect skin carefully and change position frequently.
- Maintain appropriate clothing to protect against drafts.
- Teach patient to recognise signs and symptoms.

Objectives of management

The objectives of management of the acutely spinal cord injured patient are to prevent further damage, treat the neurological injury, realign the spine and prevent and/or treat complications. Depending on the level of neurological deficit and associated injuries, the patient may require admission to the ICU. The role of immediate surgical intervention is limited. Impingement of spinal nerves from injuries, such as facet dislocation or cauda equina syndrome, requires emergency surgery. However, studies from the 1960s and 1970s have shown no improvement with emergency surgical decompression, except in the case of extradural lesions, such as epidural haematomas or abscesses. Patients with acute spinal cord injury are best treated, once stabilised, at a regional spinal cord injury centre such as QENSIC, to provide ongoing definitive care.

Examination

As with all trauma patients the primary survey should focus on life-threatening conditions. Assessment of airway, breathing and circulation takes precedence and the spinal cord injury must be considered concurrently. Clinical evaluation of a patient with suspected spinal cord injury must focus on symptoms related to the vertebral column (most commonly pain) and any motor or sensory deficits. Ascertaining the mechanism of injury is also important in identifying the potential for spinal injury.

The spinal cord is divided into 31 segments, each with a pair of anterior (motor) and dorsal (sensory) spinal nerve roots. On each side, the anterior and dorsal nerve roots combine to form the spinal nerve as it exits from the vertebral column through the neuroforamina. The spinal cord extends from the base of the skull and terminates near the lower margin of the L1 vertebral body. Thereafter, the spinal canal contains the lumbar, sacral and coccygeal spinal nerves that comprise the cauda equina. Therefore, injuries below L1 are not considered spinal cord injuries since they involve the segmental spinal nerves and/or cauda equina. Spinal injuries proximal to L1, above the termination of the spinal cord, often involve a combination of spinal cord lesions and segmental root or spinal nerve injuries.

The dorsal columns are ascending sensory tracts that transmit light touch, proprioception and vibration information to the sensory cortex. They do not decussate until they reach the medulla. The lateral spinothalamic tracts transmit pain and temperature sensation. These tracts usually decussate within three segments of their origin as they ascend. The anterior spinothalamic tract transmits light touch. Autonomic function traverses within the anterior interomedial tract. Sympathetic nervous system fibres exit the spinal cord between C7 and L1, while parasympathetic system pathways exit between S2 and S4.

Injury to the corticospinal tract or dorsal columns, respectively, results in ipsilateral paralysis or loss of sensation to light touch, proprioception and vibration. In contrast to injuries of the other tracts, injury to the lateral spinothalamic tract causes contralateral loss of pain and temperature sensation. Because the anterior spinothalamic tract also transmits light touch information, injury to the dorsal columns may result in complete loss of vibration sensation and proprioception but only partial loss of light touch sensation. Anterior cord injury causes paralysis and incomplete loss of light touch sensation. In the anterior interomedial tract, higher spinal cord lesions cause increasing degrees of autonomic dysfunction.

The American Spinal Injury Association (ASIA) has established standard neurological definitions to classify spinal cord injury (Figure 4.1). Neurological injury is the lowest (most caudal) level with normal sensory and motor function. For example, a patient with C5 quadriplegia has, by definition, abnormal motor and sensory function from C6 down. Assessment of sensory function helps to identify the different pathways for light touch, proprioception, vibration and pain. Differentiating a nerve root injury from a true spinal cord injury can be difficult. If neurological deficits suggest multilevel involvement, spinal cord injury rather than a nerve root injury is probable. In the absence of spinal shock, motor weakness with intact reflexes indicates an injury to the spinal cord, while motor weakness with absent reflexes indicates a nerve root lesion. In all patients assessment of deep tendon reflexes and perineal evaluation is critical. The presence or absence of sacral sparing is a key prognostic indicator. The sacral roots may be evaluated by documenting reflexes as shown in Box 4.2.

Box 4.2 Evaluation of sacral roots

- Perineal sensation to light touch and pinprick
- Bulbocavernous reflex (S3 or S4)
- Anal wink (S5)
- Rectal tone
- Urine retention or incontinence
- Priapism

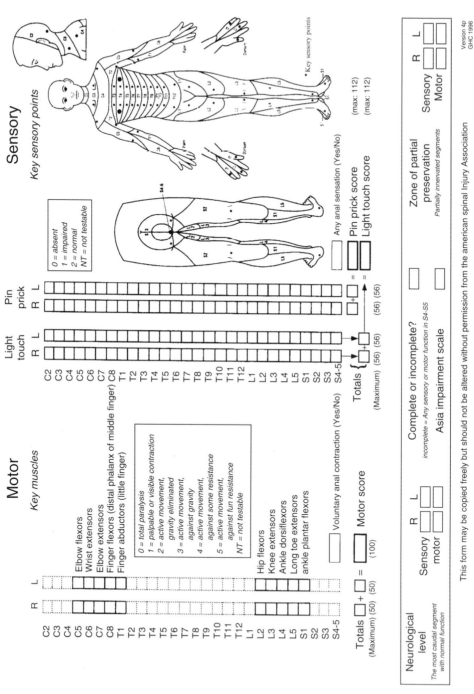

Figure 4.1 American Spinal Injury Association (ASIA) Standard Neurological Classification of spinal cord injury.

Primary and secondary spinal cord injury

Initial mechanical trauma includes traction and compression forces. Direct compression of neural elements by fractured and displaced bone fragments, disc material and ligaments injures both the central and peripheral nervous systems. Blood vessels can be damaged, axons disrupted, neural-cell membranes broken and microhaemorrhages can occur. The spinal cord may swell causing secondary ischaemia which results when the swelling exceeds venous blood pressure. Autoregulation of blood flow ceases, and spinal neurogenic shock leads to systemic hypotension, thus exacerbating ischaemia. Ischaemia, release of toxic chemicals from disrupted neural membranes, and electrolyte shifts trigger a secondary injury cascade that has marked detrimental effects on top of the initial mechanical damage.

Primary spinal cord injury can arise from mechanical disruption, transection, extradural pathology or distraction of neural elements, and usually occurs with fracture and/or dislocation of the spine. However, primary spinal cord injury may also occur in the absence of spinal fracture or dislocation, e.g. due to penetrating injuries such as gunshot wounds. More commonly, displaced bony fragments can cause penetrating spinal cord or segmental spinal nerve injuries. In children, primary spinal cord injury without spinal fracture or dislocation may result from longitudinal distraction with or without flexion and/or extension of the vertebral column. The spinal cord is tethered more securely than the vertebral column and spinal cord injury may present without radiological abnormality.

The major causes of secondary spinal cord injury are vascular injury to the spinal cord caused by arterial disruption, arterial thrombosis, or hypoperfusion due to shock. This hypoperfusion slows or blocks action potentials along axons, contributing to spinal shock. In addition, damaged cells, axons and blood vessels release a variety of cytotoxic substances. Glutamate floods out of injured spinal neurones, axons and astrocytes, overexciting neighbouring neurones, which results in a huge influx of calcium ions that trigger free radical release culminating in neuronal cells death. Excitotoxicity affects myelin-producing oligodendrocytes as well as neurones, through interaction with α-amino-3-hydroxy-5-methyl-4-isoxazole propionic acid (AMPA) receptors. This may explain why unsevered axons become demyelinated after spinal cord trauma. Studies in animals suggest that compounds that can protect cells from excess glutamate can modulate loss of myelin, e.g. selective AMPA-type glutamate receptor inhibitors [1].

Apoptosis, or programmed cell death [2], has also been shown to be involved in secondary deterioration after spinal injury. Days or weeks after the initial trauma, apoptosis may delete oligodendrocytes, affecting as many as four segments from the trauma site. Animal studies have shown that inhibition of apoptosis limits manifestations of damage after traumatic spinal cord injury [3].

The spinal cord injury must be classified as one of the cord syndromes, i.e. concussion, complete or incomplete. The incomplete cord syndromes may have variable neurological findings:

- Anterior cord syndrome involves variable loss of motor function and pain and/or temperature sensation, with preservation of proprioception.
- Brown–Séquard syndrome involves a relatively greater ipsilateral loss of proprioception and motor function, with contralateral loss of pain and temperature sensation.
- Central cord syndrome usually involves a cervical lesion, with greater motor weakness in the upper extremities than in the lower extremities. The pattern of motor weakness shows greater distal involvement in the affected extremity than proximal muscle weakness. Sensory loss is variable, and the patient is more likely to lose pain and/or temperature sensation than proprioception and/or vibration. Dysesthesias, especially those in the upper extremities (e.g. sensation of burning in the hands or arms), are common. Sacral sensory sparing usually exists.
- Conus medullaris syndrome is a sacral cord injury with or without involvement of the lumbar nerve roots. This syndrome is characterised by areflexia in the bladder, bowel and, to a lesser degree, lower limbs. Motor and sensory loss in the lower limbs is variable.
- Cauda equina syndrome involves injury to the lumbosacral nerve roots and is characterised by an areflexic bowel and/or bladder, with variable motor and sensory loss in the lower limbs. Since this syndrome is a nerve root injury rather than a true spinal cord injury, the affected limbs are areflexic. This injury usually is caused by a central lumbar disk herniation.

Shock

Spinal or neurogenic shock can be defined as the complete loss of all neurological function, including reflexes and rectal tone, below a specific level. It is associated with autonomic dysfunction and refers to loss of haemodynamic stability with hypotension, bradycardia, hypothermia and peripheral vasodilatation resulting from the interruption of sympathetic nervous system control in acute spinal cord injury. It usually does not occur with spinal cord injuries below the level of T6, and shock associated with these lower thoracic spine injuries should be considered haemorrhagic until proven otherwise.

The blood supply of the spinal cord consists of the anterior and posterior spinal arteries. The anterior spinal artery supplies the anterior two-thirds of the cord, and ischaemic injury to this vessel results in dysfunction of the corticospinal, lateral spinothalamic and autonomic interomedial pathways. Anterior spinal artery syndrome involves paraplegia, loss of pain and temperature sensation, and autonomic dysfunction. The posterior spinal arteries primarily supply the dorsal columns. The anterior and posterior spinal arteries arise from the vertebral arteries in the neck and descend from the base of the skull. Various radicular arteries branch off the thoracic and abdominal aorta to provide collateral flow. It is important to remember that vascular injury may cause a cord lesion at a level several segments higher than the level of spinal injury. For example, a lower cervical spine fracture may result in disruption of the vertebral artery that ascends through the affected vertebra and the resulting vascular injury may cause an ischaemic high cervical cord injury. Cervical hyperextension injuries may cause ischaemic injury to the central part of the cord, causing a central cord syndrome.

Haemorrhagic shock may be difficult to diagnose because history-taking and physical examination may be limited by autonomic dysfunction. Disruption of autonomic pathways prevents tachycardia and peripheral vasoconstriction that normally characterises shock, and occult internal injuries with associated haemorrhage may be missed. In all patients with suspected spinal cord injury and hypotension, a search for sources of bleeding should be made before hypotension is attributed to neurogenic shock, and indeed shock may be both neurogenic and haemorrhagic. When the injury is above T6, tachycardia and peripheral vasoconstriction may not be present. When hypotension occurs in a spinal fracture without neurological deficit, it is probably due to haemorrhage.

Treatment

The ultimate goal of therapy for patients with spinal cord injury is to improve motor function and sensation.

Methylprednisolone

Management of acute spinal cord injuries has included the use of steroids for the past 30 years. Mechanical injury to the spinal cord initiates a cascade of secondary events such as ischaemia, inflammation and calcium-mediated cell injury [4]. Methylprednisolone has neuroprotective effects in animal studies, via inhibition of lipid peroxidation and calcium influx and through its anti-inflammatory effects. Three well-designed, large, randomised clinical trials (National Acute Spinal Cord Injury Studies – NASCIS I, II and III) were undertaken to investigate the effect of steroid administration in patients with acute spinal cord injury [5–7]. NASCIS I examined the change in motor function in specific muscles and changes in light touch and pinprick sensation from baseline. The study detected no benefit from methylprednisolone, but the dose was considered to be below the therapeutic threshold determined from animal experiments. NASCIS II therefore used a much higher dose, and patients were randomly assigned to receive a 24 h infusion of methylprednisolone, naloxone or placebo within 12 h after acute spinal cord injury. Again, there was no benefit overall in the methylprednisolone group but, *post hoc* analyses revealed a small increase in the total motor and sensory score in a subgroup of patients who had received the drug within 8 h after injury. Despite the questionable validity of such a *post hoc* analysis, 24 h, high-dose methylprednisolone infusion started within 8 h after injury became an implied standard of care.

Subsequent clinical trials have provided conflicting evidence about steroid treatment in acute spinal cord injury. A Japanese study attempted to replicate the results seen in the 8 h subgroup from NASCIS II and reported improved function at 6 months in a larger number of muscles and sensory dermatomes among subjects who received high-dose methylprednisolone infusion than among those who received only low doses of the drug or no drug [8]. However, the study lacked detail about randomisation and outcome measures, and it included only 74% of the enrolled subjects in the outcome analysis. Another, underpowered, prospective, randomised trial that used a methylprednisolone regimen similar to that used in NASCIS II found no improvement in motor and sensory scores at 1 year [9].

The third study, NASCIS III, compared a 48-h infusion of methylprednisolone with a 24 h infusion started within 8 h after injury and found no benefit from extending the infusion beyond 24 h [7]. Again, only *post hoc* analyses showed a benefit from extending the infusion to 48 h when treatment was started between 3 and 8 h after injury. No other study has verified the primary outcome of 48 h versus 24 h or the *post hoc* conclusion of benefit from starting treatment between 3 and 8 h after injury. A Cochrane Review meta-analysis of all of the NASCIS trials and the Japanese study concluded that 24 h, high-dose methylprednisolone infusion within 8 h after spinal cord injury is effective [10]. The controversy about the *post hoc* analyses of NASCIS data continues and sadly subsequent studies have lacked the rigour to clarify the situation.

Although methylprednisolone is accepted as the standard of care, despite equivocal evidence, steroid therapy is not without risk. Many acute spinal cord injured patients are critically ill, have polytrauma, have impaired lung capacity and are vulnerable to infection. The incidence of sepsis and pneumonia was higher in patients who received high-dose methylprednisolone in all of the NASCIS studies and other smaller studies, although the differences were only significant in NASCIS III [7]. Hyperglycaemia and gastrointestinal complications were also reported following high-dose methylprednisolone treatment. Methylprednisolone may be harmful, particularly if infusion goes beyond 24 h [11]. However, increased strength in one or more muscles below a spinal segment is important for patients with cervical spinal cord injuries and even a small improvement may be beneficial.

In some countries there is a recommendation that "a high-dose, 24 h infusion of methylprednisolone started within 8 h after an acute closed spinal cord injury is not a standard treatment or a guideline for treatment but, rather, a treatment *option*, for which there is very weak level II and III evidence".

Traction

Although clinicians have been aware of the concept of traction for many centuries, it was not used as a therapeutic option until the late 18th century. At that time, the primary indications for spinal traction were the correction of scoliosis and spinal deformity, the management of rickets, and for relieving backache of any origin or location. Later in the 19th century, attempts were made to treat a multitude of neurological disorders with spinal traction (including conditions such as Parkinson's disease and impotence). By the first half of the 20th century, the accepted uses of spinal traction became primarily focused in the areas of cervical spine surgery and, more frequently, in the management of spinal trauma and pain.

Instability is defined as damage to the cervical spinal column, either through trauma or disease, resulting in a potential for movement or misalignment of fractured bones prior to healing or abnormal movement of the injured region with a likelihood of additional neurological damage. Traction is an extremely effective means of realigning a cervical spinal dislocation and providing stabilisation for these types of cervical spine injury.

Spinal traction provides longitudinal force to the axis of the spinal column. In other words, parts of the spinal column are "pulled" in opposite directions in order to stabilise or change the position of damaged aspects of the spine. The force is usually applied to the skull through a series of weights or a fixation device and requires that the patient is either kept in bed or placed in a halo vest. Throughout the middle of the 20th century, hooks or tongs that were firmly attached to the skull were used. The main complication from the use of skull tongs was a possibility for penetration of the skull by the pins used to attach the tongs to the head. A solution to this problem appeared in the early 1980s through an advance known as the Gardner–Wells tongs. For patients requiring long-term treatment, the halo vest is preferentially used over the Gardner–Wells tongs and bed-based traction. The halo brace is also often used as the initial treatment for odontoid fractures (located at the second cervical vertebrae of the neck).

Neurological deterioration has been reported in patients with cervical disc dislocations undergoing traction and reduction, attributed to the high incidence of disc herniations in patients with facet dislocations. This has prompted the use of magnetic resonance imaging (MRI) scanning prior to reduction of cervical spine using traction. Other large studies have refuted this showing no neurological deterioration in reduction in awake and co-operative patients. An MRI should always be obtained if the patient is unco-operative or will require reduction under anaesthesia. If the scan demonstrates a disc herniation, an anterior discectomy and fusion may be required prior to reduction.

Surgery

The goals of any surgical intervention are to reduce fractures and dislocation, to stabilise injured segments and to decompress the neural elements. Ligament injuries in the spine are potentially unstable and are best treated surgically. In a patient with neurological deficit secondary to a spinal injury who also has an upper thoracic injury, surgical stabilisation will enable early mobilisation and thus avoid pulmonary complications. Surgery to allow decompression and so prevent further deterioration is also required in patients with progressive neurological deficits who have radiological evidence of compression of either the cord or cauda. Open spine fractures should follow similar guidelines for compound fracture management in the long bones.

There remain two main controversies concerning surgical treatment: the timing of surgery and the choice of surgical approach (anterior or posterior). Early surgical stabilisation of the spine in trauma patients raised some concerns including aggravation of pulmonary decompensation by prone positioning, blood loss incurred by spinal surgery and possibility that occult injuries, especially to the intra-abdominal viscera, may be masked by early surgical intervention.

Early surgical intervention is based on experimental studies in dogs, which showed benefits of early decompression in reversing cord injuries [12]. Surgical treatment in patients with complete motor and sensory paraplegia has no influence on prognosis. Early internal stabilisation surgery has practical advantages in terms of rehabilitation compared with external (halo) stabilisation devices. Important advances have been made in the past decade in surgical procedures and hardware for internal spine stabilisation.

There are advantages to both anterior and posterior approaches to surgery after acute spinal trauma. A review of literature does not show a distinct advantage of one approach over the other. There is lower morbidity and less potential for disturbance of the vascular supply to an already injured cord using a posterior approach, whereas anterior surgery allows more thorough canal clearance in patients with significant canal compromise.

Promotion of cell regeneration

Axons in mature mammals undergo little spontaneous regeneration (reviewed by Selzter [13]). For spinal cord regeneration, electrical transmission via neurones, oligodendrocytes and adequately myelinated large-calibre axons, with the involvement of astrocytes, must take place. Myelin function can be enhanced by improvement of transmission through partly demyelinated axons, increasing of remyelination by surviving oligodendrocytes, or replacement of oligodendrocytes. Axonal regeneration can be aided by blockage of inhibitory molecules such as myelin-associated neurite growth inhibitors, with specific antibodies promotion of axonal growth with neurotrophic factors. However, axons need to be directed to appropriate targets with "guidance molecules" (netrins, cell-adhesion molecules, specific matrix proteins). Studies in rats suggested that combining multiple nerve bridges with fibrin tissue glue impregnated with acidic fibroblast growth factor and an elaborate orthopaedic manoeuvre to assist in apposition of the cut ends of the spinal cord result in greater regeneration of axon tracts and improved functional recovery [14]. Although these findings have not been reproduced in other laboratories, more than 50 patients with spinal cord injury have received peripheral nerve grafts but no results have been published.

Replacement of cells

Various studies in animals have suggested that transplantation of embryonic spinal cord results in the incorporation of cells into the injured spinal cord, resulting in a degree of functional recovery, particularly in neonatal animals or if the spinal cord was not completely transected [15]. Success has also been achieved in animals by transplantation of stem cells isolated from the spinal cord, or embryonic stem cells. Macrophages and other immune cells that accumulate in the central nervous system after injury release cytokines, which inhibit axon growth and increase the synthesis of inhibitory proteoglycans that prevent regeneration. Local injection of autologous macrophages has been claimed to be useful.

Complications

An injury to the spinal cord is a dynamic process and the full extent of injury may not be immediately apparent. Incomplete cord lesions may evolve into more complete lesions and, more commonly, the injury level may rise during the hours to days after the initial event, despite optimal treatment. A complex cascade of pathophysiological events accounts for this clinical deterioration. One of the first signs of neurological deterioration is the extension of the sensory deficit and a repeat neurological examination may reveal that the sensory level has risen one or two segments. Repeat neurological examinations to check for progression are essential.

Pressure sores

Careful and frequent turning of the patient is required to prevent pressure sores, and denervated skin is particularly prone to this complication. This can be done through the use of a special selection of beds such as the turning frames of Stryker/Foster or the Rotorest bed. Some of these beds such as the Rotorest bed can allow application of traction in various planes. The patients should be removed from the backboard as soon as possible. Many patients have stable vertebral fractures and yet still spend hours on a hard backboard unnecessarily.

Pulmonary problems

Pulmonary complications are common after spinal cord injury. There is a direct correlation between pulmonary complications and mortality and both are related to the level of neurological injury. The clinical assessment of respiratory function must include careful history-taking regarding respiratory complaints and underlying cardiopulmonary co-morbidity such as chronic obstructive pulmonary disease or heart failure. Respiratory rate, chest wall expansion, abdominal wall movement, cough, and chest wall and/or pulmonary injuries must be evaluated. Diagnosis of hypoxia or carbon dioxide retention may be difficult. The degree of respiratory dysfunction is ultimately dependent on the presence of any pre-existing pulmonary co-morbidity, the level of the spinal cord injury and any chest wall or lung injury. There may be loss of ventilatory muscle function from denervation and/or associated chest wall and lung injury, such as pneumothorax and haemothorax, or pulmonary contusion may also contribute. There may be decreased central ventilatory drive as a result of head injury or alcohol and drugs. In addition, there is a direct relationship between the level of cord injury and the degree of respiratory dysfunction. With high lesions (i.e. C1 or C2), vital capacity is only 5–10% of normal, and cough is absent. With lesions at C3–C6, vital capacity is 20% of normal, and cough is weak and ineffective. With high thoracic cord injuries (i.e. T2, T3, T4), vital capacity is 30–50% of normal, and cough is weak. Lower cord injuries have little impact on respiratory function, such that respiratory dysfunction is minimal in injuries at T11 with essentially normal vital capacity and strong cough. There may be other findings suggesting respiratory dysfunction including agitation, anxiety, or restlessness, poor chest wall expansion, decreased air entry, rales, rhonchi, pallor, cyanosis, increased heart rate, paradoxical movement of the chest wall, increased accessory muscle use and moist cough.

The incidence of deep vein thrombosis (DVT) in patients with spinal cord injury has been reported as between 15% and 100% with an incidence of pulmonary emboli of around 5% in these patients, and an associated mortality of 3–5%. Prophylaxis with heparin should be used unless contra-indicated.

Pulmonary oedema may occur as a result of aggressive fluid administration during the resuscitation phase but other causes are also important. The use of invasive cardiovascular monitoring to guide the administration of fluids, especially during spinal shock, where haemodynamic changes such as hypotension and bradycardia occur due to loss of sympathetic nervous system function, is valuable. Glucose-containing fluid may aggravate neurological injury. Neurogenic pulmonary oedema may occur in some spinal cord injuries where protein-rich alveolar fluid leaks from pulmonary capillaries, due to a transient but marked increase in sympathetic activity associated with the trauma (see Chapter 2). The pathogenesis of the oedema is incompletely understood, but may be due to hypoxia-mediated increased pulmonary vascular permeability.

Rigorous pulmonary hygiene protocols include frequent position change, incentive spirometry, chest percussion, assisted coughing and tracheal suctioning. Bradycardia and, in some instances, cardiac arrest during suctioning of patients with cervical spinal cord injury has been reported, due to predominant parasympathetic autonomic activity. Concomitant hypoxia seems to be a further predisposing factor for this exaggerated vasovagal response during tracheal suctioning.

Aspiration

Patients with cervical spinal cord injury are prone to aspiration of stomach contents. In traumatic spinal cord injury patients may have full stomachs from recent food or alcohol ingestion, altered mental status, impaired airway reflexes and gastric stasis resulting in increased risk of aspiration of gastric contents; the incidence of gastric aspiration in trauma victims with spinal injury may be as high as 38%.

Early respiratory consequences of gastric aspiration such as respiratory failure, bronchospasm, chemical pneumonitis, bacterial pneumonitis and acute respiratory distress syndrome (ARDS) may occur, but aspiration can also decrease gastric volume and the potential risk of aspirating gastric contents; however, it may also induce vomiting, leading to increased intracranial pressure.

The management of patients with aspiration of gastric contents depends on the severity of respiratory dysfunction and may include ventilation with positive end-expiratory pressure (PEEP). Steroids after aspiration have no effect on outcome and may result in pulmonary abscess, and prophylactic antibiotic treatment is not recommended.

Prognosis

Patients with a complete spinal cord injury have a less than 5% chance of recovery. If complete paralysis is present 72 h after injury, recovery is essentially zero. The prognosis is much better for the incomplete cord syndromes. If some sensory function remains, there is a more than 50% chance that the patient will eventually be able to walk. Ultimately, 90% of patients who have a spinal cord injury return to their homes and regain independence. Providing an accurate prognosis for the patient with an acute spinal cord injury is not possible in the acute stages and is best avoided. In the early 20th century, the mortality rate 1 year after injury in patients with complete lesions approached 100%. Much of the improvement since then can be attributed to the introduction of antibiotics to treat pneumonia and urinary tract infection. Currently, the 5-year survival rate for patients with traumatic quadriplegia exceeds 90%.

The best predictor of improved outcome is retention of sacral sensation (S4–S5), especially pinprick, between 72 h and 1 week after injury. Many patients may regain one level of motor function within 6 months after injury. Age contributes to prognosis, with patients under the age of 50 years showing better recovery than older patients. Clinical examination is still the best way to assess prognosis.

Summary

The objectives of management of the acutely spinal cord injured patient are to prevent further damage, treat the neurological injury, realign the spine and prevent and/or treat complications. Depending on the level of neurological deficit and associated injuries, the patient may require admission to the ICU before transfer to a regional spinal injuries centre.

References

1 Beattie MS, Hermann GE, Rogers RC, Bresnahan JC. Cell death in models of spinal cord injury. *Prog Brain Res* 2002;**137**:37–47.
2 Webster NR. Apoptosis and the inflammatory process. In Galley HF, ed. *Critical Care Focus 10: Inflammation and Immunity*, London: BMJ Books, 2003, pp. 18–32.
3 Carlson GD, Gorden C. Current developments in spinal cord injury research. *Spine J* 2002;**2**:116–28.
4 Green BA, Kahn T, Klose KJ. A comparative study of steroid therapy in acute experimental spinal cord injury. *Surg Neurol* 1980;**13**:91–7.
5 Bracken MB, Shepard MJ, Hellenbrand KG, Collins WF, Leo LS, Freeman DF *et al.* Methylprednisolone and neurological function 1 year after spinal cord injury. Results of the National Acute Spinal Cord Injury Study. *J Neurosurg* 1985;**63**:704–13.
6 Bracken MB, Shepard MJ, Collins WF, Holford TR, Young W, Baskin DS *et al.* A randomized, controlled trial of methylprednisolone or naloxone in the treatment of acute spinal cord injury. Results of the Second National Acute Spinal Cord Injury Study. *N Engl J Med* 1990;**322**:1405–11.

7 Bracken MB, Shepard MJ, Holford TR, Leo-Summers L, Aldrich EF, Fazl M *et al*. Administration of methylprednisolone for 24 or 48 hours or tirilazad mesylate for 48 hours in the treatment of acute spinal cord injury. Results of the Third National Acute Spinal Cord Injury Randomized Controlled Trial. National Acute Spinal Cord Injury Study. *JAMA* 1997;**277**:1597–604.

8 Otani K, Abe H, Kadoya S, Nakagawa H, Ikata T, Tominaga S *et al*. Beneficial effect of methylprednisolone sodium succinate in the treatment of acute spinal cord injury. *Sekitsui Sekizui J* 1996;**7**:633–47.

9 Petitjean ME, Pointillart V, Dixmerias F, Wiart L, Sztark F, Lassie P *et al*. Medical treatment of spinal cord injury in the acute stage. *Ann Fr Anesth Reanim* 1998;**17**:114–22.

10 Bracken MB. Pharmacological intervention for acute spinal cord injury [Cochrane review]. In *The Cochrane Library*: Issue 1, 2001. Oxford: Update Software.

11 Hurlbert RJ. Methylprednisolone for acute spinal cord injury: an inappropriate standard of care. *J Neurosurg* 2000;**93**:1–7.

12 Delamarter RB, Sherman J, Carr JB. Pathophysiology of spinal cord injury. Recovery after immediate and delayed decompression. *J Bone Joint Surg Am* 1995;**77**:1042–9.

13 Selzer ME. Promotion of axonal regeneration in the injured CNS. *Lancet Neurol* 2003;**2**:157–66.

14 Cheng H, Cao Y, Olson L. Spinal cord repair in adult paraplegic rats: partial restoration of hind limb function. *Science* 1996;**273**:510–13.

15 Tessler A, Fischer I, Giszter S, Himes BT, Miya D, Mori F, Murray M. Embryonic spinal cord transplants enhance locomotor performance in spinalized newborn rats. *Adv Neurol* 1997;**72**:291–303.

5: Rationale for direct brain cooling after head injury

PETER ANDREWS

Introduction

In the search for ways to improve outcome after brain injury, temperature and methods of manipulating it for therapeutic purposes has been the subject of considerable research effort. Systemic and head selective hypothermia have both been shown to convey neuroprotection after brain injury in animals. However, a trial of systemic hypothermia in human traumatic brain injury did not improve outcome at 6 months. Suppression of immune response and increase in infection are recognised side-effects of systemic hypothermia. However, pyrexia is common in humans after a severe neurological insult and even mild pyrexia has a detrimental effect on the compromised brain. Given this, and the risks and difficulties associated with systemic hypothermia, reducing pyrexia after brain injury may be appropriate. This article describes the physiological mechanisms of selective brain cooling and reviews current evidence of benefit.

Pyrexia and the compromised brain

Epidemiological evidence suggests that pyrexia is extremely common after brain injury. In Edinburgh we found that almost 90% of the patients with acute traumatic brain injury had pyrexia at some point during their intensive care unit (ICU) stay and that there was a relationship between the pyrexia and functional recovery of the brain [1]. Kilpatrick et al. [2] investigated fever in neurosurgical patients admitted to the ICU using a common definition of rectal temperature >38.5°C. Of the 428 patients studied 47% had a febrile episode. Fever is therefore common in brain injury patients and hyperthermia may worsen the neurological injury. Treatment of fever is a clinical issue that requires better management. Reith et al. [3] examined the relationship between body temperature on admission and various indices of stroke severity and outcome in 390 patients with acute stroke and found that mortality was lower and outcome better in the patients with only mild hyperthermia on admission. Body temperature was independently related to initial stroke severity, infarct size, mortality and outcome in survivors. For each 1°C increase in body temperature the relative risk of poor outcome rose by 2.2 (95% CI 1.4–3.5) ($p < 0.002$). These data suggest that, in acute ischaemic stroke, an association exists between body temperature and outcome. However, only an intervention trial of hypothermic treatment can prove whether this relation is associated or causal. Clearly the risk of patients not recovering independence is important on health-economic grounds. These studies certainly suggest a role for the management of temperature in brain-injured patients.

Clinical relevance

Small variations in brain temperature can determine the extent of histopathological injury in animal models of brain injury. Whereas mild hypothermia protects the brain from ischaemic and traumatic brain injury, mild hyperthermia can worsen outcome. Selective brain cooling has many advantages over whole body cooling, including the elimination of harmful side-effects, such as cardiac arrhythmias. Potential mechanisms by which mild hyperthermia is detrimental are thought to include increased metabolic demand for oxygen, excitatory neurotransmitter traffic and cellular acidosis.

The increased work that nose breathing requires compared to oral breathing suggests that nose breathing may be physiologically important. Brain cooling would certainly be physiological justification for the extra work. Nose breathing is more work for infants than adults and yet they prefer to use nose breathing instead of mouth breathing. Selective brain cooling may explain why nose breathing is so important to infants despite the work it requires. Du Boulay et al. [4] suggest that selective brain cooling might be the explanatory link between pyrexia, prone position and heavy wrapping as risk factors for sudden infant death syndrome (SIDS). This would also explain why mouth breathing increases the risk of SIDS and dummy use reduces it.

Nasal airflow may have subtle but significant effects that are important to the brain, which may be particularly relevant in ventilated patients who breathe through an endotracheal tube or tracheostomy. In such severely ill patients, even small improvements in physiology can make an additive difference and may present an argument for restoring nasal airflow in these patients as soon as possible [5].

Possible mechanisms for pyrexia after brain injury

There are several mechanisms by which fever or pyrexia could lead to a worse outcome after brain injury. We know that a rise in temperature results in a rise in intracranial pressure, which can potentially reduce brain perfusion and increase the requirement for oxygen, and since oxygen delivery may be compromised due to hypotension, this may worsen the brain injury. Some years ago the excitatory amino acid glutamate was found to be directly toxic to neuronal cell cultures [6]. More recently, Suehiro et al. [7] provided evidence that small variations in brain temperature are able to modify glutamate excitotoxicity. The results also suggested that the change in glutamate diffusion in the extracellular space is one mechanism by which mild hypothermia and hyperthermia exert their protective and harmful effects respectively.

An effect of temperature on the inflammatory response has been shown in many forms of acute brain injury. The immune system and the central nervous system are functionally connected and interact with one another in response to infection or trauma; an array of systemic responses begins, i.e. acute-phase proteinemia, neutrophilic leucocytosis, changes in the circulating levels of various hormones, and fever. It is now generally recognised that many of these responses are modulated by the brain. It has recently been proposed that immune signals are transported to the brain by peripheral nerves, predominantly the vagus. The macrophages of the liver (Kupfer cells) start producing small amounts of cytokines in response to their activation, coupled into a complex with the already pre-activated anaphylatoxic component of complement. These cytokines can immediately activate adjacent sensory paraganglia of the hepatic vagus nerve, which carries these stimuli to the nucleus tractus solitarius, which in turn sends them out to the hypothalamus via the ascending noradrenergic pathways. This fast avenue of communication between the immune system and the brain is activated not only in pathological situations, corresponding to fever, but is also an important component of systemic homeostasis, e.g. regulation of body temperature.

A study by Chatzipanteli et al. [8] used myeloperoxidase as a marker of polymorphonuclear leucocyte accumulation in relation to temperature after experimental traumatic spinal cord injury in rats. They showed that hypothermia reduced the degree of inflammation as shown by reduced myeloperoxidase activity and hence reduced leucocyte infiltration. The results of this study suggest a potential mechanism by which hypothermia improves outcome following spinal cord injury. So again modulation of temperature might beneficially affect the neuroinflammatory process.

The effects of mild hypothermia on oedema and expression of c-fos and heat shock protein (hsp70) messenger ribonucleic acid (mRNA) were examined during acute focal cerebral ischaemia in rats subjected to middle cerebral artery occlusion under either normothermia ($37.5\,^{\circ}$C) or hypothermia ($33\,^{\circ}$C) [9]. Magnetic resonance imaging (MRI) was used to monitor changes in the apparent diffusion coefficient of water (ADC) throughout the ischaemic period. ADC is simply a measure of the diffusion of water; if the oedema is extracellular and extravascular, it has a high diffusion coefficient and if it is intracellular, it has a low diffusion coefficient. The results showed that the size of the region with reduced ADC was smaller during hypothermia than during normothermia. Expression of both c-fos and hsp70 mRNA were markedly reduced by hypothermia. Transient ADC reduction and c-fos expression are associated with spreading neurodepression, which is believed to contribute to lesion expansion during acute focal ischaemia. The results suggest that part of the neuroprotective effect of hypothermia may be due to a reduced incidence of "spreading depression". Even mild hypothermia reduced acute phase and immediate–early gene expression, the amount of oedema by MRI perfusion, both of which are implicated in the neuroinflammatory response after trauma.

Traumatic brain injury is also associated with arachidonate release and may be associated with an imbalance of vasoconstricting and vasodilating cyclo-oxygenase metabolites, which tends to promote thrombogenesis and vasoconstriction. In the small study by Aibiki et al. [10], the levels of thromboxane B2 (TXB2) and 6-keto prostaglandin F1α (6-keto PGF1α) were measured in arterial and internal jugular bulb blood from 26 patients with traumatic brain injury. Patients were randomised into either of two groups: a hypothermic group ($n = 15$), in which the patients were cooled to 32–33°C and a normothermic group ($n = 11$), in which the patients' body temperature was controlled at 36–37°C by surface cooling using the same treatment as the hypothermic group. Body temperature control including normothermia was started 3–4 h after injury and lasted for 3–4 days, after which the patients were rewarmed at a rate of approximately 1°C/day. Arterial TXB2 levels on admission in both groups were high, but not 6-keto PGF1α, thereby causing an imbalance of the prostanoids after injury. In the normothermic group, TXB2 decreased transiently but increased again 3 days after injury. In the hypothermic group, such differences disappeared shortly after therapy. Hypothermia attenuated differences in TXB2 levels between arterial and internal jugular bulb blood, which may reflect reduced cerebral prostanoid production. The Glasgow Outcome Scale score 6 months after the insult was significantly higher in the hypothermic group than that in the normothermic group. The results suggest that moderate hypothermia may reduce prostanoid production after brain injury and minimise imbalance of TBXA2 and prostaglandin I2.

Systemic hypothermia after brain injury

Despite these small studies suggesting a benefit of hypothermia after brain injury, a recent clinical trial of moderate hypothermia in traumatic brain injury was stopped early because of lack of effect of induction of moderate hypothermia [11]. Hypothermia (33°C) was initiated randomly within 6 h of injury in 392 patients with coma after closed head injury and maintained for 48 h by means of surface cooling, or normothermia (37°C). All patients otherwise received standard treatment. The outcome was poor (defined as severe disability, a vegetative state, or death) in 57% of the patients in both groups. Mortality was similar in both groups (28% and 27% respectively). The patients in the hypothermia group had a longer hospital stay than those in the normothermia group, but fewer patients in the hypothermia group had raised intracranial pressure than those in the normothermia group. The authors concluded that treatment with hypothermia, with the body temperature reaching 33°C within 8 h after injury, was ineffective in improving outcomes in patients with severe brain injury (Table 5.1).

Although this was very disappointing given the experimental evidence supporting hypothermia after brain injury, there are several potential reasons for these results. Firstly, the control group were maintained at 37°C, which we know from epidemiological data is not "normal" after brain injury. The untreated patient population have a fever, such that the control group in this study also effectively had a therapeutic intervention to reduce their core temperature. Secondly, there may have been poor management of the diuresis commonly associated with hypothermia, with decreased serum magnesium, phosphate, potassium and calcium. All of these can cause severe systemic upset, but importantly loss of total body magnesium has been associated with a worse outcome from head injury. Rats overloaded with magnesium have a significant difference in their functional brain recovery following traumatic brain injury.

Although pyrexia after brain injury is common and detrimental, systemic hypothermia seems to convey little benefit and increases morbidity from infection. Thus the concept of direct brain cooling has arisen. Experimental research supports the concept of "cool brain–warm body" to confer cerebral protection [5].

Direct brain cooling

Physiological brain cooling mechanisms

In general, the arterial blood perfusing the brain is cooled through the systemic venous blood returning to the heart, where the cool venous blood from the body surface (nasal mucosa, scalp) heat exchanges in a counter-current mechanism with the cerebral arterial circulation. In some species, such as cats, dogs, sheep and goats, there is a mechanism for selective brain cooling in which the carotid blood supply to the brain is thermally conditioned prior to entering the circle of Willis. Countercurrent heat exchange is achieved by a network of fine vessels (called the carotid rete) in contact with cranial venous plexuses and lakes receiving cool venous blood from the systemic heat exchangers of the head. The carotid rete is connected to the

Table 5.1 Body temperature on admission and outcome six months after severe brain injury in patients treated with induction of hypothermia or normothermia

Treatment Group	Number with body temperature ≤ 35.0°C on admission	Number (%) with poor outcome*	Relative risk (95% CI)†	p value	Number with body temperature > 35.0°C on admission	Number (%) with poor outcome*	Relative risk (95% CI)†	p value
All patients‡	102		0.8 (0.6–1.0)	0.09	264		1.1 (0.8–1.3)	0.7
Hypothermia	62	38 (61)			127	69 (54)		
Normothermia	40	31 (78)			137	71 (52)		
Patients ≤ 45 years old	81		0.7 (0.5–1.0)	0.02	233		1.0 (0.8–1.3)	0.84
Hypothermia	48	25 (52)			115	59 (51)		
Normothermia	33	25 (76)			118	59 (50)		
Patients > 45 years old	21		1.1 (0.8–1.5)	0.60	31		1.3 (0.9–2.0)	0.23
Hypothermia	14	13 (93)			12	10 (83)		
Normothermia	7	6 (86)			19	12 (63)		

*Poor outcome was defined as severe disability, vegetative state or death, and was adjusted for age and Glasgow coma score on admission.
†Values indicate the relative risk in the hypothermia group as compared with the normothermia group. CI denotes confidence interval.
‡Data are presented for 366 patients because temperature on admission was missing for two patients, outcome data were missing for seven patients, and Glasgow coma score on admission, age, or both were missing for 17 patients.
From Clifton et al (11) with permission

circle of Willis through a short anastomotic artery. Within the carotid rete–venous plexus (i.e. a selective heat exchanger), heat from the warmer arterial blood is transferred to the cooler venous blood returning from heat-dissipating systemic heat exchangers of the head. Conversely, vertebral artery blood is not thermally conditioned by a countercurrent heat exchange mechanism and enters the circle of Willis at the same temperature as the blood leaving the aortic arch. The difference between vertebral blood temperature (systemic cooling only) and carotid blood temperature (systemic and selective cooling) is determined primarily by the heat loss from the carotid rete and is a good indicator of selective brain cooling. Another mechanism for selective brain cooling, found in species that do not have the carotid rete (e.g. humans, rabbit and rat), is via conductive heat loss from the scalp.

The study by Einer-Jensen and Khoorooshi [12] showed that an animal species without a rete mirabile is able to decrease the brain temperature through nasal airflow. In their study, temperatures were measured continuously in 11 rats via two thermometers, one inserted into the brain and the other into the rectum. The nasal cavities were flushed with oxygen (250–1000 ml/min) for 15-min periods, interrupted by 15-min control periods. The mean brain temperature decreased by $0.43 +/- 0.03°C$ with individual values up to $1.11°C$ during the flushing periods. The decrease was oxygen-flow dependent, but did not correlate with rectal temperature, suggesting that the cooling was related to the blood flow. Assuming that these findings can be extended to man – also without rete mirabile – this suggests that brain temperature can be decreased by nasal flushing with air or oxygen in intubated patients with hyperthermia. This simple treatment may reduce hyperthermia and be beneficial after head injury, trauma or brain ischaemia.

Direct brain cooling in man

There are three mechanisms that are thought to be involved in selective brain cooling in man. The first is cooling of venous blood by the skin, which cools the arterial (carotid) blood supply to the brain. The second is cooling through heat loss through the skull. The third is through evaporation from upper airways. Evaporation from scalp and face and secretions from the nose cool blood in emissary, diploic, ophthalmic and facial veins. The dura mater transmits the cooling to the cerebrospinal fluid, which influences parenchymal temperature by both direct contact, and via arteries extending within the subarachnoid space, the pial vascular network and the parenchyma. The cavernous sinus is also thought to be involved in brain cooling by countercurrent heat exchange with the internal carotid artery. Selective brain cooling by heat loss through skull and upper airways is anatomically complementary and results in the brain being almost completely encircled with cool venous blood and cool air.

In terms of temperature transfer from the inner brain, however, convection is more important than conduction. Blood from the face flows into the intracranium through the ophthalmic veins when human subjects become hyperthermic. Hirashita et al. [13] investigated a possible mechanism underlying this change in direction of flow. Five volunteers underwent either passive body warming or exercise in a climatic chamber at 28°C and 40% relative humidity. During both tests, forehead sweat rate and skin blood flow started to increase shortly upon warming. The ophthalmic vein blood flow began to change, such that the venous blood flowed from the face into the intracranium significantly later. The skin blood flow and mean body blood flow at flow reversal was significantly higher during passive body warming than during exercise. The authors concluded that the mechanism for switching the direction of ophthalmic blood flow was triggered by a high temperature in the brain and not by thermal input from the periphery of the body.

The superior sagittal and cavernous sinuses receive venous drainage from the nose. Proximity of the carotid artery to the trachea, larynx and pharynx is important and in effect the nose may be more important for temperature regulation than respiration. Nasal heat loss by both evaporation and convection can account for over 10% of body heat loss in humans. In addition, convective heat loss results from air turbulence and flow resistance caused by the nose. In a study of intracranial temperature in conscious patients during and after an upper respiratory bypass, Mariak et al. [14] measured temperatures subdurally between the frontal lobes and cribriform plate, and on the vault of the skull in four subjects. Further measurements were also made in the oesophagus and on the tympanic membrane. Restoration of airflow in the upper respiratory tract under conditions of mild hyperthermia gave a rapid drop in subdural temperature. In three patients the intracranial temperature at the basal aspect of the frontal lobes fell below the oesophageal temperature. Thus the study showed local selective cooling of the brain surface below that of the trunk temperature. Intensive breathing by the patients afterwards produced a cooling at the site of subdural temperature measurement at a rate of up to 0.1°C/min. The results suggested that cooling of the upper airway could directly influence human brain temperature.

White et al. [15] also demonstrated that nasal mucosal blood flow increases in response to skin warming and rises in core temperature. Five subjects wearing only shorts and a thick felt hat with ear flaps were immersed to the neck in a bath at 40°C. Tympanic, oesophageal, mean skin, nose skin and ear pinna skin temperatures were recorded at 1-min intervals. Nasal mucosal blood flow on the lower septal wall was estimated using a laser Doppler flow meter. At rest both tympanic and oesophageal temperatures were 36.5°C, but tympanic temperature dropped significantly below the oesophageal temperature during body warming, despite impeded heat loss from the head due to the hat. Tympanic and oesophageal temperature increased to 37.3°C and 37.5°C respectively during the immersion and all skin temperatures remained steady or increased. Body warming significantly increased nasal mucosal blood flow by approximately three times from resting values by the end of immersion. During the period of increasing core temperatures nasal mucosal blood flow was significantly correlated to tympanic and oesophageal temperatures, suggesting the blood flow change was a thermoregulatory response. The increased nasal mucosal blood flow during hyperthermia supports the hypothesis of respiratory cooling involvement in selective brain cooling of humans.

To identify the temperature differences in readings taken from the brain, jugular bulb and core in head-injured patients, Rumana et al. [16] studied 30 patients with severe head injuries who had measurements of brain and core body temperatures (Figure 5.1). In 14 patients jugular venous blood at the level of the jugular bulb was also measured. Brain temperature increased by a mean of 1.1°C (range 0.30–2.1°C) over the core body temperature. Jugular vein and core body temperatures were similar suggesting that jugular vein temperature measurement is not a good measurement of brain temperature. The difference in the brain and body temperatures increased when cerebral perfusion pressure decreased to between 20 and 50 mmHg. The difference in the brain and body temperatures decreased in those patients treated with barbiturate coma. The authors concluded that direct measurement of temperature in head-injured

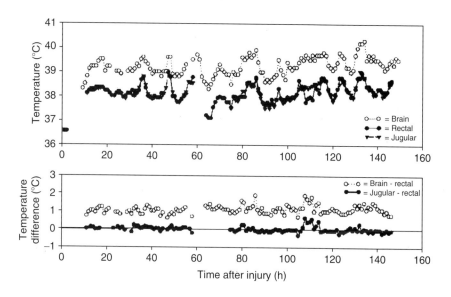

Figure 5.1 Example of changes in brain, rectal and jugular blub temperatures over time. Brain temperature is around 1.0°C (1.8°F) higher than both rectal and jugular temperatures during the first 5 days after injury in 30 patients with severe head injuries. From Rumana et al. Crit Care Med 1998 [16], with permission.

patients is a safe procedure. Temperatures in the brain were typically higher than core body temperature and jugular bulb temperature. These findings support the potential importance of monitoring brain temperature and the importance of controlling fever in severely head-injured patients since brain temperature may be higher than expected.

It is worth noting, however, that if the immune response to body temperature is modulated by the brain, making the brain alone hypothermic may cause immune depression and increase the risk of infection. In addition, if immune defence is accelerated and more efficient at raised temperatures, reducing brain temperature to normal in fever may increase morbidity and mortality from infection.

Conclusion

In addition to brain cooling by arterial blood, humans have mechanisms for selective blood cooling – the reduction of brain temperature below arterial core trunk temperature by heat loss from the skull and upper airways. This has clinical relevance for SIDS and brain injury.

References

1 Jones PA, Andrews PJ, Midgley S, Anderson SI, Piper IR, Tocher JL, Housley AM, Corrie JA, Slattery J, Dearden NM et al. Measuring the burden of secondary insults in head-injured patients during intensive care. *J Neurosurg Anesthesiol* 1994;**6**:4–14.
2 Kilpatrick MM, Lowry DW, Firlik AD, Yonas H, Marion DW. Hyperthermia in the neurosurgical intensive care unit. *Neurosurgery* 2000;**47**:850–5.
3 Reith J, Jorgensen HS, Pedersen PM, Nakayama H, Raaschou HO, Jeppesen LL, Olsen TS. Body temperature in acute stroke: relation to stroke severity, infarct size, mortality, and outcome. *Lancet* 1996;**347**:422–5.
4 du Boulay GH, Lawton M, Wallis A. The story of the internal carotid artery of mammals: from Galen to sudden infant death syndrome. *Neuroradiology* 1998;**40**:697–703.
5 Andrews PJD, Harris BA. The rationale for selective brain cooling. In Vincent JL, ed. *Year Book of Intensive Care & Emergency Medicine*. Berlin, Heidelbrg, New York: Springer-Verlag, 2002, pp. 738–47.
6 Choi DW, Maulucci-Gedde M, Kriegstein AR. Glutamate neurotoxicity in cortical cell culture. *J Neurosci* 1987;**7**:357–68.
7 Suehiro E, Fujisawa H, Ito H, Ishikawa T, Maekawa T. Brain temperature modifies glutamate neurotoxicity in vivo. *J Neurotrauma* 1999;**16**:285–97.
8 Chatzipanteli K, Yanagawa Y, Marcillo AE, Kraydieh S, Yezierski RP, Dietrich WD. Posttraumatic hypothermia reduces polymorphonuclear leukocyte accumulation following spinal cord injury in rats. *J Neurotrauma* 2000;**17**:321–32.
9 Mancuso A, Derugin N, Hara K, Sharp FR, Weinstein PR. Mild hypothermia decreases the incidence of transient ADC reduction detected with diffusion MRI and expression of c-fos and hsp70 mRNA during acute focal ischemia in rats. *Brain Res* 2000;**887**:34–45.

10 Aibiki M, Maekawa S, Yokono S. Moderate hypothermia improves imbalances of thromboxane A2 and prostaglandin I2 production after traumatic brain injury in humans. *Crit Care Med* 2000;**28**:3902–6.

11 Clifton GL, Miller ER, Choi SC, Levin HS, McCauley S, Smith KR Jr, Muizelaar JP, Wagner FC Jr, Marion DW, Luerssen TG, Chesnut RM, Schwartz M. Lack of effect of induction of hypothermia after acute brain injury. *N Engl J Med* 2001;**344**:556–63.

12 Einer-Jensen N, Khorooshi MH. Cooling of the brain through oxygen flushing of the nasal cavities in intubated rats: an alternative model for treatment of brain injury. *Exp Brain Res* 2000;**130**:244–7.

13 Hirashita M, Shido O, Tanabe M. Blood flow through the ophthalmic veins during exercise in humans. *Eur J Appl Physiol Occup Physiol* 1992;**64**:92–7.

14 Mariak Z, White MD, Lewko J, Lyson T, Piekarski P. Direct cooling of the human brain by heat loss from the upper respiratory tract. *J Appl Physiol* 1999;**87**:1609–13.

15 White MD, Cabanac M. Nasal mucosal vasodilatation in response to passive hyperthermia in humans. *Eur J Appl Physiol Occup Physiol* 1995;**70**:207–12.

16 Rumana CS, Gopinath SP, Uzura M, Valadka AB, Robertson CS. Brain temperature exceeds systemic temperature in head-injured patients. *Crit Care Med* 1998;**26**:562–7.

6: The role and value of imaging in acute spinal trauma

EVELYN TEASDALE

Introduction

Imaging has a central role in the diagnosis, assessment and on-going management of patients with spinal trauma. No radiographs are required in an asymptomatic fully conscious, sober patient with no other serious distracting injury and no spinal pain. The widespread availability of computed tomography (CT) and magnetic resonance imaging (MRI) has had a dramatic impact on spinal imaging.

The role of imaging in suspected spinal trauma is to identify and define any major bony injury and assess the stability of that injury to identify any other injuries, spinal or otherwise, to identify soft tissue injury and to exclude any reversible compressive lesion. Prognostic information may also be offered if required. Stability is the fundamental issue in spinal trauma because if the fracture is unstable, neurological damage is possible. Stability is dependent on the integrity of intervertebral discs, facet joints and ligaments of the spine. Stability can be defined as the ability to maintain normal alignment of the spine, provide support for the head and torso and protect the neural elements – all under normal physiological stresses.

Epidemiology of spinal injury

Approximately 20 people per million injure their spinal cord in the UK each year. Around 700/year are complete cord injuries and 700/year are incomplete. Spinal cord injuries can happen to anyone, at any age although they are most common in men aged between 16 and 30 (Figure 6.1). Almost 50% of all spinal cord injuries occur in a motor vehicle accident, 20% from a fall, 15% from some act of violence and 14% from a sports-related accident (Figure 6.2). The commonest sports for spinal injury is perhaps unsurprisingly, diving. The accidents that cause many spinal cord injuries are related to drug or alcohol abuse. Trauma to the spine and spinal

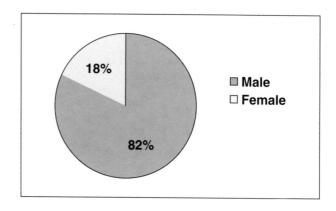

Age at time of injury	Percentage
76–90	1.0
61–75	4.4
46–60	9.2
31–45	19.4
16–30	61.1
0–15	4.9

Figure 6.1 Age and sex distribution of spinal injury.

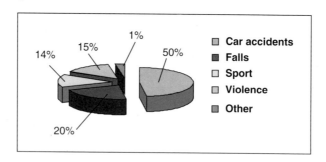

Figure 6.2 The majority of spinal injuries arise from road traffic accidents.

cord is a significant cause of disability. In the western world the yearly incidence of disability related to spinal trauma can be estimated at about 5 per 100 000 people. The most frequent neurological deficit is incomplete tetraplegia (30.6%), followed by complete paraplegia (25.8%), complete tetraplegia (22.1%) and incomplete paraplegia (19.3%). Since nearly 60% of cases occur in young adults aged between 16 and 30 years, spinal injury carries a significant cost in terms of lifetime care and loss of productivity.

Conformation of suspected spinal injury is found in 2–6% of patients using plain x-ray film examination. The greater the degree of mobility of the spine, the greater the chance of injury: 66% of injuries are cervical with thoracic injuries being the least common. Roughly 20% of patients with spinal fracture will have another injury at a different spinal level.

The cord lesion may result from anatomical disruption, compression, ischaemia, or any combination of these factors. From a practical point of view active compression requiring acute surgery needs to be distinguished from spinal injury secondary to contusion or concussion with complete recovery of the spinal axis. Spinal injury can occur as a result of hyperflexion or rotation, vertical compression, hyperextension with or without rotation and lateral flexion plus others (shown in Table 6.1).

Denis' three-column principle

The degree of stability of spinal injury is based upon the Denis three-column principle: the spine is unstable and will undergo further deformation and cord damage if two of the three (vertebral body, pedicle or neural arch) columns are fractured (Figure 6.3).

In a retrospective study of 412 thoracolumbar injuries, Denis introduced the concept of middle column or middle osteoligamentous complex between the traditionally recognised posterior ligamentous complex and the anterior longitudinal ligament [1]. This middle column is formed by the posterior wall of the vertebral body, the posterior longitudinal ligament and posterior annulus fibrosus. The third column appears crucial, as the mode of its failure correlates both with the type of spinal fracture and with its neurological injury. In this study, spinal injuries were assessed as minor and major. Minor injuries included fractures of transverse processes, facets, pars interarticularis, and spinous processes. Major spinal injuries were further classified into four different categories: (1) compression fractures, (2) burst fractures, (3) seat-belt-type injuries and (4) fracture dislocations. They were then divided into subtypes demonstrating the very wide spectrums of these four conditions.

The three-column model proposed by Denis predicted the biomechanical stability of the vertebral–ligamentous complex in response to fracture or injury and the subsequent need for treatment with active immobilisation or fixation. The model was derived from morphological characteristics of each fracture and then refined to reflect CT scan findings consistent with

Table 6.1 Types of spinal injury

Type of injury	Examples
Hyperflexion	Anterior subluxation (hyperflexion sprain) Bilateral interfacetal dislocation (BID) Simple wedge (compression) fracture Clay Shoveler's fracture Flexion teardrop fracture
Hyperflexion/rotation	Unilateral interfacetal dislocation (UID)
Hyperextension	Hyperextension dislocation Avulsion fracture of the anterior arch of the atlas Fracture of the posterior arch of the atlas Extension teardrop fracture Laminar fracture Traumatic spondylolisthesis ("hangman's" fracture)
Hyperextension/rotation	Pillar fracture Pedicolaminar fracture-separation
Vertical compression	Jefferson's bursting fracture, C1 Burst (bursting, dispersion, axial loading) fracture, lower cervical spine
Lateral flexion	Unilateral occipital condylar fracture Unilateral fracture, lateral mass, C1 Uncinate process fracture Transverse process fracture
Other	Occipito-atlantal dissociation 　Subluxation 　Dislocation Odontoid fractures Torticollis (atlanto-axial rotary displacement or fixation) Atlanto-axial rotary dissociation 　Subluxation 　Dislocation

each fracture type. The three-column model modified an earlier model, which suggested that disruption of the posterior ligamentous complex only was needed to infer biomechanical instability. Instability with the three-column concept recognises that at least two of the three columns must be disrupted to create an unstable fracture. This predictive model has been used in conjunction with injury forces and mechanisms of injury producing fracture to classify all vertebral fractures into four major categories.

Stable injuries can be summarised as having no potential for impingement or injury to the spinal cord, no potential for displacement of the fracture during the healing process and no displacement as a result of normal physiological stresses after healing (Boxes 6.1 and 6.2).

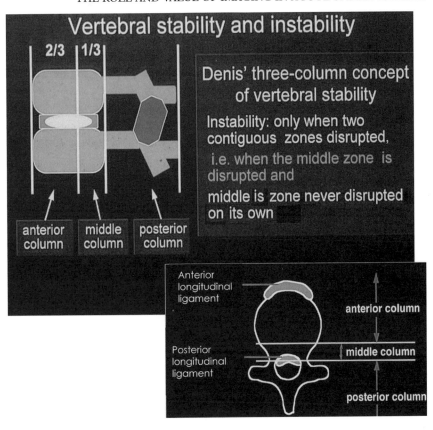

Figure 6.3 The three-column model of stability[1].

Common types of injury

Hyperflexion injuries occur through distraction of posterior elements and compression of the anterior column. Anterior subluxation or hyperflexion sprain is the classic "whiplash" injury resulting from abrupt deceleration, e.g. running your car into a stationary car. It results in posterior ligament complex injury and the posterior annulus fibrosis and disc can be disrupted. The injury is initially stable but there is a 21–50% incidence of delayed instability. Bilateral interfacetal dislocation is a soft tissue injury resulting in disruption to the anterior and posterior longitudinal ligament (ALL and PLL respectively). There is a high risk of cord damage and this injury is unstable. A simple wedge compression occurs in the mid to lower cervical spine and results in an impacted superior endplate, with no vertical fracture and the ALL and disc remain intact. Although the injury is initially stable, there is a risk of delayed instability if the post-ligament

67

Box 6.1 Stable and unstable spinal injuries

Stable injuries
- Vertebral components will not be displaced by normal movement.
- An undamaged spinal cord is not in danger.
- There is no development of incapacitating deformity or pain.

Unstable injuries
- Further displacement of the injury may occur.
- Loss of 50% of vertebral height.
- Angulation of thoracolumbar junction of $>20°$.
- Failure of at least two of Denis' three columns.
- Compression fractures of three sequential vertebrae can lead to post-traumatic kyphosis.

---

complex is injured and does not heal. A flexion teardrop fracture is the most devastating cervical spine injury compatible with life. There is severe flexion with disruption of all ligaments and of the disc with vertebral facture. The injury is unstable.

Hyperflexion injury with rotation results in dislocation of the facet joint opposite the direction of rotation, with disruption of the posterior ligament complex and articular joint capsule. The ALL, disc and PLL remain intact. This injury is most common at C5–6 and C6–7 and is stable unless a fracture isolates the articular process.

Box 6.2 Examples of stable and unstable spinal injuries

Unstable
- Bilateral interfacetal dislocation (BID)
- Flexion teardrop
- Unilateral interfacetal dislocation (UID) + fracture
- Jefferson's fracture
- Hangman's Dens (high) extension teardrop (in extension)

Stable
- Anterior subluxation
- Simple wedge
- Clay Shoveler's fracture
- Laminar
- Pillar
- UID
- Simple burst
- Atlas arch fracture

Hyperextension injuries include traumatic spondylolisthesis or "Hangman's fracture", hyperextension dislocation, anterior arch avulsion of the atlas, posterior arch fracture of the atlas, extension teardrop fracture and laminar fracture. Hangman's fracture represents 4–7% of all cervical fractures and/or dislocations and is the most frequent fracture in fatal traffic accidents. Hyperextension dislocation is a soft tissue injury with disruption of ALL, disc and PLL. There is compression of cord anteriorly by the vertebral body and posteriorly by ligaments, resulting in a paralysed patient with "normal" cervical spine. Spondylosis is a predisposing factor and this injury is unstable. The injury is often associated with facial injuries and diffuse soft-tissue swelling with normally aligned vertebrae on lateral radiograph. In addition, the acute central cervical cord syndrome occurs, with haemorrhage into central cord with a range of symptoms from upper extremity paralysis to quadriplegia.

An atlas anterior arch avulsion is a hyperextension injury due to intact longus colli muscles and atlanto-axial ligaments with a transverse fracture to the mid or inferior arch and no neurological deficit. The injury is stable. An atlas posterior arch fracture is from compression of the arch between the occiput and spinous process of C2, with fractures through both sides of the arch, from the posterior to the lateral masses. The injury is stable. An extension teardrop fracture is visible as a triangular fragment from the anterior inferior corner of the vertebral body. It is most common in elderly patients with osteopenia and is unstable in extension, but stable in flexion. A laminar fracture is a posterior arch fracture of a lower cervical vertebra as it is compressed between the superior and inferior vertebral lamina. Fragments are often displaced into the spinal canal. This is a stable injury.

Injuries caused by hyperextension with rotation are the results of upward force on the forehead or upper face with the head rotated resulting in pillar fracture (a vertical fracture of the articular pillar from impaction by the superior articular mass), or pedicolaminar fracture through the ipsilateral pedicle and lamina resulting in a free-floating lateral mass. If the latter fracture extends into the foramen transversarium, vertebral artery injury is possible. This injury is unstable if associated with contralateral interfacetal dislocation.

Vertical compression or axial load injury occurs as the result of force delivered to top of skull through the occipital condyles to the cervical spine at the instant that the cervical spine is straight. The resulting injuries are Jefferson fractures and burst fractures. The Jefferson fracture results in splitting of the C1 ring with fracture of both the anterior and posterior arch and may result from a single break in each arch (anterior and posterior). It can be bilateral or unilateral. Half of Jefferson fractures are associated with other fractures. There is no neurological deficit but the fracture is unstable. Burst fractures occur commonly at C3–C7, and it is presumed that the compressed disc bulges into inferior endplate causing the vertebral body to explode from the inside. There is usually association with injury to spinal canal but the ALL, disc and posterior column are usually intact and the injury is stable.

Complete spinal cord injury

Complete spinal cord injury results in loss of all motor and sensory function below the level of the injury, and is typified by bilateral external rotation of the legs, loss of pain, temperature, vibration sensation, loss of bowel and bladder function. Spinal or neurogenic shock may develop. In comparison, acute anterior cord syndrome results in complete paralysis and hypesthesia and hypalgesia to the level of the injury, but there is preservation of touch, motion, position and vibration sense.

Assessment of spinal injury (Box 6.3)

Plain radiographs

Hoffman et al. [2] reported a study on 1000 consecutive patients with blunt trauma. Clinicians completed data forms for each patient before x-ray results were known, including mechanism of injury, evidence of intoxication, presence of cervical spine pain and/or tenderness, level of alertness, presence of focal neurological deficits, and other severely painful injuries unrelated to the cervical spine. An estimation of the likelihood of cervical spine injury was also made. Of the 974 patients for whom data forms were completed, 27 had cervical spine fractures. All of these had at least one of the following four characteristics: midline neck tenderness, evidence of intoxication, altered level of alertness, or a severely painful injury elsewhere. The authors concluded that cervical spine radiology may not be necessary in patients without tenderness in the neck, intoxication, altered level of alertness, or other severely painful injury. A follow-up study by Hoffman et al. [3] of over 34 000 patients suggested five clinical criteria that could predict low risk for spinal injury after blunt trauma, called the National Emergency X-Radiography Utilization Study (NEXUS) criteria.

The exclusion of cervical injury on clinical grounds is reliable provided the patient is alert, has not consumed alcohol or other intoxicants and no neck signs, relevant neurological deficits or distracting injuries are present. The acronym NSAID is used to select patients for cervical spine x-ray (Box 6.4). This takes into account any focal deficit upon neurological examination, any tenderness posterior of the midline of the spine, the degree of alertness, evidence of intoxication and any other painful injury that might distract the patient from the pain of the spinal injury. Clinical examination alone can reliably assess all blunt trauma patients who are

---

Box 6.3 Clinical management of suspected spinal injury

History

- Strongly suspect spinal injury if any major accident, unconscious patient, fall from a height, sudden jerk of neck after rear end car collision, facial injuries or head injury.
- Ask about neck or back pain, numbness, tingling, weakness, ability to pass urine.

Examination

- Logroll – look for bruising, palpate for a step, tenderness.
- Repeated neurological examination to determine neurological damage and its progression/resolution.
- Thorough overall examination for fractures, etc. as patient may not feel pain.

Imaging

- X-rays – cervical spine AP, lateral including C7/T1, open mouth view of odontoid. Swimmer's view or pull arms down. AP and lateral view of other tender areas of spine.
- CT scan shows bony injury.
- MRI shows soft tissue involvement.

If neurological damage

- Catheterise.
- Note reduced blood pressure and bradycardia due to neurogenic shock (temporary generalised sympathectomy). Rule out hypotension due to haemorrhage elsewhere. May need treatment with vasopressors, not fluid resuscitation.
- Invasive monitoring required.
- Give methylprednisolone i.v. 30 mg/kg over 15 min then 5.4 mg/kg/h for next 23 h. Needs to be given within 8 h. Discuss with the spinal team.
- Attend to skin by turning.

---

alert, non-intoxicated, and who report no neck symptoms. However, considerable discretion must be used. For instance, deeming an injury to be sufficient to distract a patient from the pain of a neck injury should be left to the judgement of the physician, as well as the level of intoxication and its effect on a patient's reliability.

Box 6.4 The NEXUS cervical spine criteria

- N   neurological examination – any deficit?
- S   spinal examination – any tenderness posterior midline of spine?
- A   alertness – any alteration?
- I   intoxication – any evidence?
- D   distracting injury – any painful injury which might distract from the pain of a spinal injury?

However, not all spinal injuries show up on x-ray. This is particularly relevant in children where the spinal cord can be damaged without any fracture of the bone being seen – spinal cord injury without radiological abnormality (SCIWORA).

Magnetic resonance imaging and computed tomography

The widespread availability of cross-sectional imaging has had a dramatic impact on spinal imaging [4–7]. Prior to CT, plain film myelography was the only means of depicting intraspinal pathology by revealing compression of the thecal sac and nerve root sleeves. CT scanning provided excellent bony imaging in cross section, but still required myelographic injection for identification of thecal sac contents. The high contrast resolution of MRI permits visualisation of the soft tissues within the spinal canal, allowing detailed assessment of most intraspinal pathology.

There is no doubt that an increasingly multislice helical CT has made a major change to our appreciation of the complexity and extent of all spinal fractures. Multiplanar and three-dimensional imaging increase understanding of the injury well beyond the base axial images. CT should be performed as a minimum from the level above the injury to the level below to determine normal anatomy for internal fixation planning if necessary: Thin sections (1 mm on the cervical region and up to 2.5 mm in the thoracic and lumbar regions) allow good base and multiplanar images using a low radiation dose technique. CT angiography can also reveal damage to blood vessels. CT is useful in confirming the efficiency of internal fixation but poor at determining if bony repair is adequate for mobilisation.

When there is clinical evidence of cord injury but no fracture is demonstrated by CT, then a dynamic flexion/extension examination should be performed when the patient is able to co-operate and is pain-free. Abnormal movement will confirm ligamentous injury requiring treatment.

Detailed comparison of MR images and histopathological examination of injured spinal cords have increased the understanding of the nature of spinal cord injuries in both the acute and chronic stages. The role of MRI is summarised in Box 6.5. Abnormalities seen on MRI explain many of the acute and progressive neurological symptoms experienced by spine-injured patients (Box 6.6).

Spinal cord injuries range from simple contusions to contusion with haemorrhagic necrosis. Simple contusions are visible on MRI as a focus of abnormal high signal intensity on T2-weighted images within the substance of the cord. This signal abnormality reflects a focal accumulation of intracellular and interstitial fluid in response to the injury. Definition is usually optimal on the midsagittal (T1- and T2-weighted images). Axial T2-weighted images offer supplementary information with regard to the involvement of structures in cross section. Oedema involves a variable length of spinal cord above and below the level of injury, with discrete boundaries

---

Box 6.5 The role of MRI

- Assess the nature of cord damage.
- Evaluate ligament and soft tissue injury.
- Offer prognostic information.
- Demonstrate vascular injury.

Box 6.6 Prognostic information from MRI findings

MRI findings	Prognosis	Points
Cord is normal	Recovery is normal	
Cord oedema	Recovery in over 50%	Minor contusion or concussion
Cord haemorrhage	No recovery	Severe contusion or haematoma
Cord compression	Variable	No correlation with prognosis
Whiplash injury	Variable	No correlation with prognosis

---

adjacent to uninvolved parenchyma. Spinal cord oedema visualised by MRI is invariably associated with some degree of spinal cord swelling.

A haemorrhagic contusion is composed of an epicentre of haemorrhage surrounded by a halo of oedema; the latter has a greater rostrocaudal extent than the central haemorrhage. Spinal cord swelling usually involves a slightly greater portion of spinal cord than oedema or haemorrhage alone. Blood degradation products produce typical paramagnetic signal abnormalities on MRI. However, the appearance of haemorrhage is time-dependent, as illustrated in Table 6.2. T1- and T2-weighted sequences are the standard sequences used in spinal trauma. As haemorrhage changes from oxyhaemoglobin to deoxyhaemoglobin over time, the signal it gives on the MR sequences changes dramatically, and both are required to adequately define the haematoma.

The detection of a sizeable focus of blood in the cord usually indicates a complete neurological injury near the haemorrhage and is commonly associated with poor neurological recovery.

However, MRI is rather too sensitive and in minor injuries such as whiplash it will demonstrate soft tissue injury in almost 50% of patients, which does not correlate with outcome and may well result in unnecessary immobilisation. In severe spinal injury MRI will define the nature of the cord injury from contusion to transection and these findings have prognostic significance. Traumatic compression by disc prolapse and extra- and subdural haematomas is uncommon but well defined by MRI, which is also useful in excluding syrinx formation in late deterioration. There are disadvantages to MRI, most notably the high scanning times, which, although they are decreasing as technology improves, are still an issue for resuscitation and safety of the patient. However, the information MRI provides is rarely required urgently.

Conclusion

The following are recommended practices: x-rays should be performed according to the NEXUS protocol, but clinical judgement should be exer-

Table 6.2 The appearance of haemorrhage on MRI is time-dependent

Time	T1	T2
0–12 h	No change/dark	No change/bright
1–7 days (acute)	No change/isointense	Dark (deoxy Hb shortens T2)
5 days to 1 month (subacute)	Bright	Dark
1–12 months (late subacute)	Bright	Bright
Months to years	Isointense	Dark

cised in the patient who complains of spinal pain – CT will surprise you with the number of unsuspected spinal fractures. A timely CT scan is worth many delayed MR images but MRI can offer good prognostic information for functional improvement.

References

1 Denis F. The three-column spine and its significance in the classification of acute thoracolumbar spinal injuries. *Spine* 1983;**8**:817–31.
2 Hoffman JR, Schriger DL, Mower W, Luo JS, Zucker M. Low-risk criteria for cervical spine radiography in blunt trauma: a prospective study. *Ann Emerg Med* 1992;**21**:1454–60.
3 Hoffman JR, Mower WR, Wolfson AB, Todd KH, Zucker MI. Validity of a set of clinical criteria to rule out injury to the cervical spine in patients with blunt trauma. National Emergency X-Radiography Utilization Study Group. *N Engl J Med* 2000;**343**:94–9.
4 Goergen S, Fong C Dalzeil K, Fennessy G. Development of an evidence-based guideline for imaging cervical spinal trauma. *Australasian Radiol* 2003;**47**:240–6.
5 Mann F, Cohen W, Linnua K, Hallam DK, Blackmore CC. Evidence-based approach to using CT in spinal trauma. *Eur J Radiol* 2003;**43**:39–48.
6 Hauser C, Visvikis G, Hinrichs C, Eber CD, Chok, Lavery RF, Livingston DH. Prospective validation of computed tomographic screening of thoracolumbar spine in trauma. *J Trauma Injury, Infect Crit Care* 2003;**55**:228–35.
7 Hollingworth W, Nathans A, Kanne J, Crandall ML, Crummy TA, Hallam DK, Wang MC, Jarvik JG. The diagnostic accuracy of computed tomography angiography for traumatic and atherosclerotic lesions of the carotid and vertebral arteries: a systematic review. *Eur J Radiol* 2003;**48**:88–102.

7: Prehospital care in trauma patients

GARETH DAVIES, DAVID LOCKEY

Introduction

Prehospital trauma care is a balance of appropriate prehospital intervention to increase the chances of survival and reduce morbidity and of timely delivery to definitive care. Information on which prehospital interventions are appropriate and who should provide them is at best scanty and often contradictory. As a result, the practice of prehospital care varies widely in all parts of the world. In the UK, the London Helicopter Emergency Medical Service delivers senior medical staff (either Consultant grade or Senior Specialist Registrar) to the scene of major trauma. It aims to provide intensive care at the roadside and deliver patients to the most appropriate hospital for their injury pattern. Elsewhere in the UK, prehospital care is delivered by ambulance technicians and paramedics, and patients are usually delivered to the nearest hospital irrespective of injury type and the resources available at the hospital.

Outside the UK there is even more marked variability in practice. In the USA and Australia the service is predominantly paramedic-delivered. In Europe prehospital care is mainly physician-led. For example, France and Germany have a comprehensive network of mobile ambulance intensive care units (ICUs) and approximately 40 helicopter air ambulances staffed by anaesthetists providing nationwide intensive care at the roadside.

The term "paramedic" covers a wide spectrum of skills, training and experience in different countries. In the USA paramedics are recruited at degree level, have thousands of hours of theoretical teaching, extensive practical training and comprehensive examination and assessment before qualification. Post qualification they have audit, recertification and medical oversight of the services they provide. In other countries such as the UK paramedics can enter technician training with school-leaver qualifications and have only 2–3 months of specific paramedic training with relatively little in the way of medical supervision and support.

Trauma epidemiology

Trauma is the leading cause of death in people aged between 1 and 35 years in the developed world. Road traffic accidents cause over 300 000 injuries, 40 000 serious injuries, and 3400 deaths a year in the UK (Box 7.1). Put into context, this is equivalent to a Lockerbie air crash monthly or a Paddington rail crash three times a week [1].

Road traffic accidents still account for the majority of deaths. In the UK the death rate from road traffic accidents has decreased substantially over the last 10 years but more recently this decline has tended to plateau. The mortality rate from road accidents in rural areas is much higher than in cities. Explanations for this difference include higher vehicle speeds and delays in alerting the medical services, in getting transport to the scene and in eventually providing transport to hospital.

Airey and Franks [2] provide a comprehensive picture of major trauma within a UK Health Region. The incidence of patients with an injury severity score of 15 or more (the definition of major trauma) was found to be 27 cases per 100 000 population (17.7/100 000 surviving to hospital). This equated to approximately one major trauma patient for every 1000 new accident and emergency (A&E) attendances. For an A&E department seeing 50 000 patients per year, this would mean approximately one multiple-injured patient per week. Similar figures have been reported by other authors [3,4].

The American College of Surgeons [5] receives 240 patients per year with an Injury Severity Score (ISS) >15 for Level One Trauma Centre accreditation and require the receiving trauma surgeons to see an average of 30 cases per year to maintain expertise. For individuals and teams in the UK the infrequency of multiple trauma has the potential to effect skill utility and performance.

The evidence base

None of the UK research funding bodies has a strategy for research into prehospital care. Literature review of the subject demonstrates less than 30

Box 7.1 Epidemiology of trauma

- Trauma is the commonest cause of death in young adults.
- An average District General Hospital will see 50–70 major trauma patients per year.
- Up to 40% of prehospital deaths may be preventable.
- Prehospital care is important but is just the start.

---

randomised studies in prehospital interventions. Since few good research studies have been carried out, practice is largely based on anecdotal experience and consensus opinion [6]. However, efforts are being made to improve this situation [7,8].

For many years the debate of prehospital care has centred around "scoop-and-run" approach versus "stay-and-stabilise" approach to care. Today there is recognition that this debate is artificial and oversimplifies the issues. The best prehospital care is probably tailored to individual cases and depends upon many factors including the type of injuries sustained, the skill base of those delivering the care and local hospital resources. For example, patients with penetrating trauma and major vascular injury are likely to benefit most by rapid transfer to hospital since advanced life support (ALS) interventions in these circumstances often only serve to delay definitive surgical treatment. In contrast, it may be better to control airway and breathing problems, and optimise oxygenation and cerebral perfusion at the accident scene prior to the transport of patients with serious head injuries. Polytrauma patients can present difficult management problems with injury patterns that have competing interests. An example of this is the head-injured patient bleeding uncontrollably from a massive pelvic injury.

The overall organisation of any trauma system may influence morbidity and mortality after injury. Considering prehospital care separately from the rest of the trauma system rather than as the start of a continuum of care is artificial. The optimal outcome of trauma patients depends on each component of the chain, from injury to rehabilitation, performing well. If patient outcome is an endpoint in the comparison between two systems of hospital care, the comparison is only valid if intensive care, surgical management, ward and rehabilitation care are all of the same standard.

The "golden hour"

The term "golden hour" is an artificial concept that is frequently used to describe the immediacy of medical care for victims of trauma, and implies that morbidity and mortality are increased if appropriate care is not available within the first hour after injury. Airey and Franks [2] reported that 35% of trauma deaths occur before reaching hospital within the first hour. A proportion of these are immediate deaths attributable to massive brain injury, direct injury to the heart, or great vessel rupture. However, others are due to potentially treatable airway, ventilation and circulation problems. Evidence from the UK suggests that up to 40% of prehospital deaths from trauma may be avoidable [9].

The time it takes to get an accident victim into hospital is easily underestimated. Often "scene times" are quoted in the literature, which often fails to take into account emergency call time, dispatch time, transport time to and from the scene and transport time from scene to ambulance. Several studies reveal that there is often a 30–45-min interval between the time of the accident and arrival at hospital even in non-trapped straightforward incidents [10–12]. A significant proportion of the "golden hour" is therefore a prehospital event. If physicians wish to deliver life-saving interventions in the first hour, they may be too late if they wait in receiving hospital for patients to arrive.

Provision of prehospital care in the UK

In the UK, doctors form part of the normal ambulance service response in only a few areas. The London Helicopter Emergency Medical Service has fulfilled this role in the capital for 15 years. However, several hospital units have operated land-based flying squads [13], and increasingly some regional helicopter air ambulances are utilising doctors on a part time basis. There is also a network of voluntary doctors (The British Association of Immediate Care Schemes) who assist ambulance services in serious cases, particularly in remote areas. Unfortunately, the organisation of these doctors is co-ordinated by local schemes and is somewhat fragmented. Skill levels are also variable.

Although the national curriculum for paramedic training does not include certain specific skills (e.g. paediatric intubation, intraosseous infusion, needle cricothyrotomy or needle thoracocentesis), some ambulance services do provide additional training for paramedics and permit their paramedics to perform these interventions. Nalbuphine, a synthetic opiate analogue without controlled drug restrictions, is often used as an analgesic but may cause problems later in hospital, because of its partial antagonist activity toward morphine.

Prehospital intubation

There are conflicting views on the role of prehospital intubation. Much of the confusion arises from the heterogenicity of the systems from which the data arise. It is presumed that intubation per se is the relevant issue, but there are many other important issues that determine the success rate of prehospital intubation and whether it is likely to be beneficial to the patient. Key issues are whether drugs are used, the skill base of the operator, the indications for intubation and the patient case mix. Often these features are not described in papers making interpretation of results difficult.

In the UK, it is usual practice for paramedics to perform non-drug-assisted tracheal intubation on trauma patients when the airway is compromised and basic airway manoeuvres have failed. Anecdotal experience shows that patients who can be intubated without the use of drugs have a poor prognosis. Lockey *et al.* [14] investigated mortality in trauma patients who were intubated before reaching hospital without anaesthetic drugs being used. This was a retrospective study using the database of a helicopter emergency medical service. This service was staffed by doctors and paramedics and was specifically targeted at trauma patients in a mainly urban area. Patients who had been intubated without drugs by either paramedics or doctors were identified and survival to hospital discharge was recorded. Although patients were attended by physicians at the scene of accident, many were intubated by ground crew paramedics before the medical team arrived. Patients were then taken to the nearest appropriate hospital by ground or air. It was found that during a 6-year period, 1480 trauma patients were intubated outside hospital and 33.2% were intubated without drugs (55.8% of these by physicians and 43.9% by paramedics). Only one of the 486 patients on whom data were available survived. This person had a cardiac arrest after penetrating chest trauma and underwent a thoracotomy at the accident scene. Fatal outcome in non-drug-assisted intubation is not surprising, since for intubation without anaesthetic drugs the patient must be profoundly unconscious. A negative association with outcome for prehospital intubation is also found in other studies [15–17]. This has led many to question the role of prehospital intubation [18,19].

One paper has found benefit from non-drug-assisted intubation. Winchell *et al.* [20] reported on the effect of prehospital tracheal intubation on outcome in patients with severe head injury in a countywide urban trauma system in the USA. Trauma patients with blunt injury and a Glasgow Coma Score <8 at the accident scene, who were transported by ground ambulance with ALS capabilities between 1 January 1991 to 31 December 1995, were included. Of the 1092 patients, 671 had severe head injury and 351 had isolated severe head injury. It was found that at the scene intubation was associated with decreased mortality from 36% to 26% in the full study group, from 57% to 36% in patients with severe head injury, and from 50% to 23% in patients with isolated severe head injury. It was concluded that prehospital tracheal intubation was associated with improved survival in patients with blunt injury and Glasgow Coma Score <8, especially in those with severe head injury.

Prehospital fluid replacement

The initiation of prehospital i.v. fluid in injured patients has been routine practice for many years. It assumed that early volume replacement in bleeding patients results in arrival at hospital in a better haemodynamic state. However, evidence from animal studies [21–24] and one human study [25] have questioned vigorous fluid replacement and suggested that a more tolerant approach to low blood pressure should be taken, an approach often termed "permissive hypotension".

Current recommendations from National Institute for Clinical Excellence [26] take account of these studies and advocate this conservative approach suggesting that fluid therapy only be administered en route to hospital and only when there is loss of a radial pulse. These guidelines also recommend the use of crystalloid, not colloid. For complex patients with both head injury and uncontrolled haemorrhage, this obviously represents a dilemma. Traditional teaching would advocate the maintenance of a good cerebral perfusion pressure and the maintenance of good systolic pressures [27]. The relative threat to the patient must be assessed and one injury given priority. Low-level evidence does exist that permissive hypotension may be applicable even in the context of head injury [28]. This is a controversial position to say the least.

The role of hypertonic saline in prehospital resuscitation is also being considered, but a recent study by Cooper *et al.* [29] suggests that there may be no advantage in its use in prehospital phase of injury, perhaps reflecting that normalisation of physiology is not advisable until bleeding is controlled or stopped.

The theory behind permissive hypotension is that restoration of blood pressure removes blood clots from surgical and non-surgical bleeding points. A natural extension of this is an effort to minimise clot disturbance by appropriate handling techniques that serve to minimise the number of times a patient is rolled. At the London Helicopter Emergency Medical Service, specific minimal handling policies are considered part of the resuscitation technique.

Summary

Prehospital care is emerging as a specialist career for doctors in Europe, Scandinavia and the USA. In Britain there are *ad hoc* local arrangements with only a small proportion of road traffic victims receiving prehospital care from a specialist doctor. Practice is largely based on experience and consensus opinion, leading to considerable variation in the delivery of medical services to trauma victims. A good practice recommendation by these authors for prehospital resuscitation is given in Box 7.2.

Box 7.2 Prehospital resuscitation

- Same principles as in hospital, but adapted to circumstances.
- Airway management can be difficult, but basic measures are important.
- Intubation without anaesthesia is unlikely to improve outcome.
- The cervical spine should be immobilised.
- Oxygen should be given.
- Haemorrhage should be controlled with direct pressure.
- If casualty is trapped ensure good venous access before release.
- Fluid resuscitation should be given to a systolic blood pressure of 90 mmHg.
- Analgesia can be achieved with Entonox or ketamine.
- Extrication requires close co-ordination between medical and fire services.
- Casualty should be "packaged for transport" with hard collar, head blocks, limb splints, scoop stretcher or vacuum mattress.
- In bleeding patients a "minimal handling policy" should be considered.

References

1 Coats TJ, Davies G. Prehospital care for road traffic casualties. *Br Med J* 2002;**324**:1135–8.
2 Airey CM, Franks AJ. Major trauma workload within an English Health Region. *Injury.* 1995 Jan;**26**:25–31.
3 Spence MT, Redmond AD, Edwards JD. Trauma audit – the use of TRISS. *Health Trends* 1988;**20**:94–7.
4 Phair IC, Barton DJ, Barnes MR, Allen MJ. Deaths following trauma: an audit of performance. *Ann R Coll Surg Engl* 1991;**73**:53–7.
5 American College of Surgeons. *Resources for the Optimal Care of Trauma Patients.* 1999.
6 Callaham M. Quantifying the scanty science of prehospital emergency care. *Ann Emerg Med* 1997;**30**:785–90.
7 Lewis RJ. Prehospital care of the multiple-injured patient: the challenge of figuring out what works. *JAMA* 2004;**291**:1382–4.
8 Sayre MR, White LJ, Brown LH, McHenry SD. National EMS Research Agenda Writing Team. The National EMS Research Agenda executive summary. Emergency Medical Services. *Ann Emerg Med* 2002;**40**:636–43.
9 Hussain L, Redmon A. Are prehospital deaths from accidental injury preventable? *Br Med J* 1994;**308**:1077–80.
10 Rainer TH, Houlihan KP, Robertson CE, Beard D, Henry JM, Gordon MW. An evaluation of paramedic activities in prehospital trauma care. *Injury* 1997;**28**:623–7.

11 Gorman DF, Teanby DN, Sinha MP, Wotherspoon J, Boot DA, Molokhia A. The epidemiology of major injuries in Mersey Region and North Wales. *Injury* 1995 Jan;**26**(1):51–4.

12 Nicholl JP, Brazier JE, Snooks HA. Effects of London helicopter emergency medical service on survival after trauma. *Br Med J* 1995;**311**:217–22.

13 Graham CA, Meyer AD. Prehospital emergency rapid sequence induction of anaesthesia. *J Accid Emerg Med* 1997;**14**:219–21.

14 Lockey D, Davies G, Coats T. Survival of trauma patients who have prehospital tracheal intubation without anaesthesia or muscle relaxants: observational study. *Br Med J* 2001;**323**:141.

15 Eckstein M, Chan L, Schneir A, Palmer R. Effect of prehospital advanced life support on outcomes of major trauma patients. *J Trauma* 2000;**48**:643–8.

16 Gausche M, Lewis RJ, Stratton SJ, Haynes BE, Gunter CS, Goodrich SM, Poore PD, McCollough MD, Henderson DP, Pratt FD & Seidel JS. Effect of out-of-hospital pediatric endotracheal intubation on survival and neurological outcome: a controlled clinical trial. *JAMA* 2000;**283**:783–90.

17 Stockinger ZT, McSwain NE. Prehospital endotracheal intubation for trauma does not improve survival over bag–valve–mask ventialtion. *J Trauma* 2004;**56**:531–6.

18 Spaite DW, Criss EA. Out of hospital rapid sequence intubation: are we helping or hurting our patients? *Ann Emerg Med* 2003;**42**:729–30.

19 Nolan J. Prehospital and resuscitative airway care: should the gold standard be reassessed? *Curr Opin Crit Care* 2001;**7**:413–21.

20 Winchell RJ, Hoyt DB. Endotracheal intubation in the field improves survival in patients with severe head injury. *Arch Surg* 1997;**132**:592–7.

21 Stern SA, Dronen SC, Birrer P, Wang X. Effect of blood pressure on hemorrhage volume and survival in a near-fatal hemorrhage model incorporating a vascular injury. *Ann Emerg Med* 1993;**22**:155–63.

22 Leppaniemi A, Soltero R, Burris D, Pikoulis E, Waasdorp C, Ratigan J, Hufnagel H, Malcolm D. Fluid resuscitation in a model of uncontrolled hemorrhage: too much too early, or too little too late? *J Trauma* 1996;**41**:439–45.

23 Smail N, Wang P, Cioffi WG, Bland KI, Chaudry IH. Resuscitation after uncontrolled venous hemorrhage: does increased resuscitation volume improve regional perfusion? *Ann Emerg Med* 1993;**22**:155–63.

24 Haizlip TM Jr, Poole GV, Falzon AL. Initial resuscitation volume in uncontrolled hemorrhage: effects on organ function. *Am Surg* 1999;**65**:215–7.

25 Bickell WH, Wall MJ Jr, Pepe PE, Martin RR, Ginger VF, Allen MK, Mattox KL. Immediate versus delayed fluid resuscitation for hypotensive patients with penetrating torso injuries. *N Engl J Med* 1994;**331**:1105–9.

26 National Institute for Clinical Excellence. *Pre-hospital Initiation of Fluid Replacement Therapy in Trauma*. London: National Institute for Clinical Excellence (NICE), 2004,p. 28.

27 The Brain Trauma Foundation. The American Association of Neurological Surgeons. The Joint Section on Neurotrauma and Critical Care: Hypotension. *J Neurotrauma* 2000;**17**:591–5.

28 Bourguignon PR, Shackford SR, Shiffer C, Nichols P, Nees AV. Delayed fluid resuscitation of head injury and uncontrolled hemorrhagic shock. *Arch Surg* 1998;**133**:390–8.

29 Cooper DJ, Myles PS, McDermott FT, Murray LJ, Laidlaw J, Cooper G, Tremayne AB, Bernard SS, Ponsford J. Prehospital hypertonic saline resuscitation of patients with hypotension and severe traumatic brain injury: a randomized controlled trial. *JAMA* 2004;**291**:1350–7.

Index